The Pediatrician's

New Baby Owner's Manual

Your Guide to the Care & Fine-Tuning of Your New Baby

D1468504

by
Horst D. Weinberg, M.D.

Quill
Driver
Books

Fresno, California

618.92
W31

Please Note:

This book is not intended to replace medical advice and should only be used to supplement regular care by your child's physician. Always consult your child's physician prior to embarking on any medical program or treatment. Every child is different, always seek professional advice when concerned.

Many of the products named in this book are trademarks. Please see trademark information, page 195.

Copyright © 1997 Horst D. Weinberg, M.D.
All rights reserved including the right of reproduction in whole or in part in any form.

Quill Driver Books titles may be purchased at special prices for educational, fund-raising, business or promotional use. Please contact:

Special Markets
Quill Driver Books/Word Dancer Press, Inc.
P.O. Box 4638, Fresno, CA 93744 • (800) 497-4909

To order an additional copy of this book please call 1- (800) 497-4909

Published by
Quill Driver Books/Word Dancer Press, Inc.
8386 North Madsen Avenue
Clovis, CA 93611
(209) 322-5917

Second printing October 1997

Weinberg, Horst D. 1928-
  The pediatrician's new baby owner's manual : your guide to the care & fine-tuning of your new baby / Horst D. Weinberg.
        p. cm.
  Includes index.
  ISBN 1-884956-07-6
  1. Pediatrics--Popular works.   I. Title.
RJ61.W3714 1996
618.92--dc20   96-35579
                                                          CIP

Printed in the United States of America

Contents

Acknowledgments

This book would not exist without the help and support of my "editor" and best friend, my wife, Carol. It was her wise advice, constant support and encouragement to continue, that helped me to finish this book against all the odds. She taught me the practical side of pediatrics.

I am indebted to the many patients who were with me over the years and from whom I learned what was important in raising their children.

And especially, thanks to my own children, David, Susan and Carla, who allowed me to practice on them during their growing-up years. They taught me that in these troubled times, it is possible to raise really nice kids, who turn into adults you can be proud of.

Introduction

After many years of practicing pediatrics and several of answering parents' questions on a weekly call-in TV program, I realized that parents have many questions that do not get answered to their satisfaction by their doctor.

This book is not to take your doctor's place. It is rather to help you, the parent, when the doctor is not immediately available, and to educate you to ask the "right" questions.

Unlike everything else that you have, your child does not come with an "instruction manual," telling you what to do or when to do it.

In the past there was the extended family: grandparents, aunts, uncles or neighbors, all available and willing to offer helpful advice. In our mobile society, many families do not live near relatives or know their neighbors and have lost this valuable resource. This lack of assistance is compounded by the fact that both parents often have to work.

However, be wary of believing everything you read on raising your child. In today's world, child-raising books based on the latest fad in parenting have become *the* source of child-care information for many parents. One can find books on anything. There are books on how to pick up your baby, how to play with your baby, and how to talk to your baby. There are also activity-a-day calendars and developmentally-correct play-groups.

Once parents begin to doubt their own intuition, they become dependent on books and specifically designed "developmental toys." Everything becomes a "lesson" and the child's play suddenly becomes hard work.

This book is designed to fill part of the void, giving you advice to help you navigate the sometimes troubled waters of parenthood without replacing you as the thinking, caring parent.

Best Advice:

There are many different ways to take care of your baby. Raise your child with your values and ideas. Use common sense. You will usually be correct. If what you do makes you and your child happy, it's probably the right thing to do.

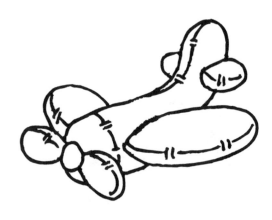

One

Preparing for Your Baby

What you will need

- ♥ A room or area for your baby to sleep in. (Babies need their own space and parents need their own bedroom.)

- ♥ A cradle or crib

- ♥ Blankets (2)

- ♥ Diapers (several dozen, cloth or disposable)

- ♥ Safety pins

- ♥ Plastic pants (4), with cloth diapers only

- ♥ Bottles (6)

- ♥ Shirts (6)

- ♥ Pacifiers (2)

- ♥ Nightgowns/sleepers (4)

- ♥ Thermometer

- ♥ Car seat

- ♥ Tylenol (acetaminophen) infant drops

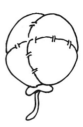

Choosing a doctor

You will need a doctor to help take care of your baby. Babies do come early, so don't wait until the last moment to pick a doctor. Together Mom and Dad should interview several pediatricians or family doctors.

Some questions you might want to ask are:

- What special training does the doctor have? (Board certification in Pediatrics or Family Practice is usually a plus.)

- Are the fees similar to what is charged in your area?

- Can you reach the doctor daytime, nights and weekends?

- Who is available when your doctor is away?

- When you call the office with a question, will you be able to talk to the doctor if you are uncomfortable with the nurse's answer?

- Does the doctor support breast-feeding or formula-feeding, depending on your interest?

- If you have a boy, will the doctor support your wishes about circumcision?

- Does the doctor prescribe antibiotics frequently or use them only if they are really needed?

- Does the office prescribe antibiotics over the telephone? (The answer should be no.)

- What is his or her level of willingness to discuss illness and treatment options with you?

Observe:

- Is the office clean and professional?

- Is the office staff friendly and helpful?

Weigh the answers you get with the observations you make and choose a doctor you are comfortable with.

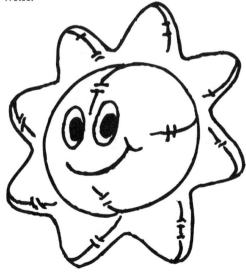

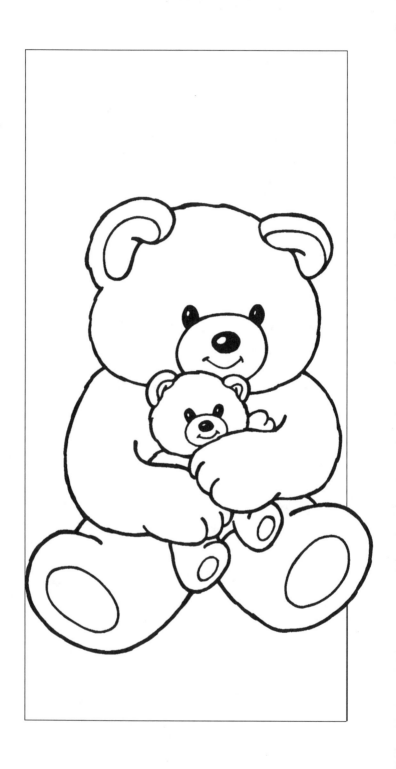

Two

Some Early Choices

Feeding: breast or bottle?

Breast feeding

It takes two to three days for the mother's body to make breast milk. During these first few days the baby gets a watery substance called colostrum, which gives your baby much needed resistance to disease. For this reason, the first few days of breast-feeding are the most important.

Most mothers can breast-feed if they want to. Breast milk looks watery, but is always the correct strength. The more your baby sucks, the more milk Mom's breasts will make.

Start breast feeding five minutes on each side and increase by one minute each feeding. Work your way up to 15 to 20 minutes on each side.

Alternate which breast you start with so that each breast gets emptied completely every other time.

Fifteen to 20 minutes on each side will empty your breasts. The baby may want to suck longer, but then you are just being a big pacifier. If you have time, that's fine, but if you have other things to do, it's OK to quit.

Some babies have a hard time latching on,

especially if the breast is engorged and the nipple does not stick out. This engorgement lasts only a few days and then your breasts will become soft and pliable again. This does not mean you have lost your milk.

If your baby has a hard time latching on, a "nipple shield," which you can buy at the drugstore, works well. The shield fits over your breast, the baby sucks on the rubber nipple of the shield and pulls your nipple into the shield. After a few days baby will have no trouble hooking on to you. (You can also use a plain rubber nipple from a baby bottle to do what the nipple shield does.)

If your baby sucks too much during the first few days of breast-feeding, your nipples may get quite sore or even crack and bleed. You cure this by cutting down the feeding time and using a nipple shield. This helps the nipples rest and heal. After a few days the nipple soreness should be gone.

Your breasts do not need special cleaning. Wash your nipples with plain water when dirty, dry them well and rub in either some vitamin E or aloe vera cream.

Mothers who are pushed by family or physician to breast-feed, but don't really want to, often are not successful at breast feeding. These mothers should consider formula-feeding.

Formula-feeding

Formula-fed babies do grow as well as

breast-fed babies. Formula can be given cold from the refrigerator and most babies will happily drink it that way.

Do not prop the bottle, but hold your baby. Contact with Mom or Dad is an important part of feeding time, for both baby and parents.

Formulas are made out of milk or soybeans. Soybean formulas may be easier to digest.

Formulas come with or without iron. The iron in iron-fortified formulas does not constipate your baby. Most babies need all the iron they can get.

There is little difference between formulas. Use what you want. Formulas come in ready-to-feed, concentrated and powder forms. Powder is the cheapest, but the most work. Ready-to-feed is expensive and the least work. Concentrated is in-between.

You can make your own good, inexpensive formula.

Mix in a one-quart container:
1 12-ounce can evaporated milk
2 tablespoons Karo syrup (corn syrup)
Fill the container to the top with water.

Light Karo will make your baby's stools firmer. Dark Karo will make your baby's stools looser.

Most babies do not need water, but it gives you something to give your child between formula- or breast-feedings.

Sterilize formula and water (boil water then cool it, or use a store-bought sterilizer) until your baby is four months of age.

From a practical standpoint, bottles and nipples are all the same. Use what you want.

Circumcision

Whether or not you have your boy baby circumcised is a personal decision. If you want to have it done, the best time is in the first two weeks of life.

Arguments for:
- Cancer of the penis is rare, but almost never occurs in circumcised males.

- There is a decrease in bladder and kidney infections in the first few years of life.

- There is probably less susceptibility to AIDS.

- There is probably less susceptibility to any sexually transmitted disease.

Arguments against:
- There is some pain.

- It costs money.

Diapers: cloth or disposable?

The purpose of the diaper is to keep your baby clean and dry.

Cloth diapers that you wash are the cheapest.

Cloth diapers washed by a diaper service are a treat.

Disposable diapers are expensive, but very convenient.

The kind of diaper you use does not make any difference; just be sure to change it when wet or dirty.

Plastic pants over the diapers are a wonderful way to protect your clothes if you use cloth diapers.

Best Advice:

Use the diapers that are convenient and easy for you. Change your baby's diapers promptly when wet or dirty!

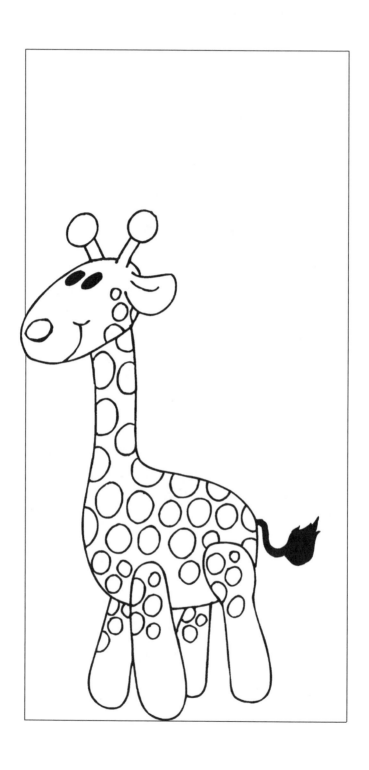

Three

A Word About Sleep— Yours and the Baby's

Yours

There are many different ways to take care of your baby. If what you do makes you and the baby happy, it's OK. Mom and Dad will get little rest for the first several weeks. Both of you will be tired and crabby. You will get to sleep again eventually, and life really *does* get better after a few months...honest.

Baby's

Babies sleep better when they do not sleep in your bedroom. Your baby needs a flat surface to sleep on, like a cradle or crib.

Babies should sleep on their side, with a blanket roll at the back for support. Try not to let your baby sleep on his or her belly. There is some question about whether sleeping on the stomach increases the frequency of Sudden Infant Death Syndrome (SIDS).

Infants sleeping on their back may have an increased risk of choking on food or mucus.

After your baby learns to roll over, how you position him or her doesn't matter. Your baby will sleep in the position in which he or she is most comfortable.

Your baby does not need a pillow, and soft pillows may be dangerous.

Get off to a good start by putting your baby down at a regular time for naps and bedtime.

When it is bedtime change and feed your baby. Put your baby down, say "Good night," and leave. If you make a habit of this from the start, your baby will be quiet and go to sleep. For the first few months, pick up and comfort your baby after a few minutes of crying.

After six to nine months of age, if your baby cries, go in and comfort him or her. Do not pick the baby up unless you need to feed or change your child. After a few days, when your baby learns that crying does not result in being picked up, he or she will stop crying at nap time or bedtime.

(See also Recommended Hours of Sleep—Infants, Children, Teenagers, page 183)

Best Advice:

Most babies do not sleep through the night for many months; they get hungry, and need food before the morning. But don't worry, both parents and baby will survive, and this ordeal gives you "bragging rights" when talking to friends and relatives.

Four

The First Year

Your baby will change a lot during the first year.

Four weeks

Most of your baby's responses are reactions to comfort or discomfort. The baby looks at people but makes no social contact. The baby's primary activities are eating and sleeping.

Four months

Your baby likes to be picked up.

Your baby follows objects with his or her eyes, coos and laughs. If you smile, baby smiles back.

Many babies roll over.

Baby starts to teethe and likes to chew on things.

Six months - nine months

Your baby likes to look around. He or she is interested in objects, holds them and moves them from hand to hand. Baby plays with his or her feet and rolls over at will; tries to crawl or creep; tries to sit up alone (often failing). Most babies smile, are sociable and can differentiate parents from strangers.

Nine months - twelve months

By one year of age babies are mobile. They creep, crawl and like to explore their environment. Many babies try to pull up to a stand and some can walk. They have eagle eyes, finding and picking up small objects with finger and thumb. Everything ends up in the mouth.

They drink from a cup, play with a spoon and want to help with their own feeding. They want to be independent, and have their own way, but are easily distracted.

Some babies now sleep through the night. Baby is aware of what goes on around him or her, is friendly and likes to socialize. Many wave bye-bye, say "Da Da" and play games like peekaboo. Some babies are fearful. They love their families but want nothing to do with strangers.

A one-year-old is mobile, boisterous, and generally fun to have around the house.

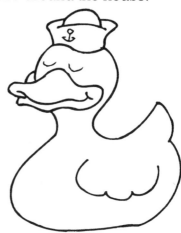

Five

Immunizations

The immunizations or "baby-shots" given in the first few years of life probably do more good for your baby than most future medical care.

They are given either by mouth or by injection, depending on the type of immunization. Injections (shots) are usually given in the upper arm, the outer thigh or the buttocks. There may be swelling, pain and redness for twenty-four to thirty-six hours where the injection was given. This is nothing to worry about. Treat this with hot compresses (a warm, wet cloth placed on the area) and baby Tylenol (acetaminophen). Do not give asprin to children under 18 years of age. (See also Fever/pain medications, page 177)

Sometimes a small, firm, non-tender lump forms at the injection site after a number of days. This also will go away by itself, but it may take several weeks or months to completely disappear. It is nothing serious; do not worry.

Immunizations your child needs:

DTP (Diphtheria, Tetanus and Pertussis)

This immunization protects your child against diphtheria, lockjaw and whooping cough. It is started at two months of age and consists of a series of three shots, each given two months apart. Boosters are necessary in the second year, on school entrance and then every ten years.

Your child may develop a fever after the shot and be a little cranky. Baby Tylenol (acetaminophen) or similar products given at the time of the shot often help to prevent this.

Don't believe any of the following common myths:

- DTP shots cause brain damage or death. There is *no* evidence to support this allegation.

- If your child misses a shot, the series must be started all over. Not true. You continue immunizations when possible.

- A tetanus shot is needed with each cut or scrape. Not true. Once a child has completed the series, a shot every ten years is all that is needed.

DTaP (Diphtheria, Tetanus, acellular-Pertussis)

This is DTP with modified acellular pertussis-material and so causes fewer, less severe reactions. It is now licensed for all ages and will probably replace DTP eventually.

Td (Tetanus full dose, Diphtheria reduced dose)

This is used after seven years of age.

Hepatitis-A

This immunization protects your child against hepatitis-A. This common cause of jaundice (yellow eyes) is spread by poor hygiene (not washing hands after going to the toilet). Most children do not get too sick, and it is not common enough for the vaccine to be routinely recommended. At the present time it is given to travelers going to Third World countries, food workers, medical workers, and workers in day-care situations where the exposure may be high. Ask your doctor about this vaccine and if your child should get it.

Hepatitis-B

The recommendations are to start this vaccine shortly after birth. There are three shots (the first at one month of age, the remaining two at five-month intervals). Boosters may be necessary later.

This vaccine is most important for teenagers and young adults who may engage in sexual activity or drug use. We give it to infants because we see babies more frequently than we see teenagers and take advantage of having them in the office to give the shots.

HIB (Meningitis)

This vaccine protects against the most common type of meningitis that can kill children in the first few years of life. It is started at two months of age, and there are two or three shots (depending on the type of vaccine your doctor uses), with a booster at fifteen to eighteen months.

DTP-HIB

This is a combination of DTP and HIB, and it saves the child from getting an extra shot. It is the ideal way to immunize your child against all four of these diseases. It is given just like the regular DTP series and does not cause any more side-effects than DTP alone.

MMR (Measles, Mumps and Rubella)

This vaccine protects your child against measles, mumps and German measles (Rubella). It is given to your baby shortly after one year of age. Your child may have a fever ten to twelve days after the shot, or even a mild rash. Treat the fever with baby Tylenol (acetaminophen). Your child is not contagious, and does not have measles.

A booster is given either on school entrance or in early teenage. Most school systems, and most colleges, now require a second MMR (booster) for admission.

Pneumovax (Pneumococcal vaccine)

This vaccine protects against the common type of bacterial pneumonias. It works quite well, but is not routinely given unless the child has been shown to have poor immunity or some chronic disease that would make him or her more susceptible. Check with your doctor.

TVOP (Trivalent Oral Polio)

This is a live (weak) virus vaccine given by mouth. It protects your child against polio (infantile paralysis). It is given at two months of age, with another set of drops two months later. A booster is necessary at twelve to eighteen months and then again at five to six years.

An injectable (killed) vaccine, IPV, is now available. The killed vaccine can be given first, followed by the live TVOP. This decreases the minimal risk of getting polio from the live vaccine and is useful for this reason when the child or a close family member has an impaired immune system.

PPD (Tuberculosis Skin Test)

This is not an immunization, but tests your child for exposure to tuberculosis. It is given at one year of age and then every one to two years.

It is a requirement for school entrance. After six years of age a PPD every two or more years is adequate.

Varivax (Chicken Pox)

This vaccine protects your child against chicken pox. It is given at or after the first birthday. Through age twelve only one shot is needed. Children thirteen years old or older and adults need two shots, four to eight weeks apart. Ask your doctor for this vaccine. Chicken pox is a miserable disease and you should protect your child from it.

What will be available in the future:

- A vaccine for rota virus. This virus causes a common form of serious diarrhea in infants.

- A vaccine for respiratory syncytial virus. This virus causes many of the colds, coughs and pneumonias in the first two years of life.

- Genetically prepared combined vaccines, giving multiple protection against various common diseases.

Six

How to Tell if Your Child is Really ill

It is important to know whether your child is really sick. Children can have many complaints and a high fever, but not be very ill or vice versa.

Here are some clues that can help you determine how sick your child is:

- Does your child respond to comforting? Can you settle him or her down easily or does crying or whining continue regardless of how hard you try to make him or her happy?

- Is your child sleepy? How easy is it to wake him or her? Does he or she remain awake or drift back into sleep?

- Does your child smile at you and interact with you, or is he or she dull or appear anxious?

- Is your child fussy, not wanting to move?

- Is your child's color normal, or is he or she pale or a little blue?

- Is your child breathing hard or grunting a little with each breath?

- Is his or her skin dry? Are his or her eyes sunken?

Any and/or all of these indicate that your child may be very sick and your doctor should be called immediately.

Best Advice:

Your own overall impression or "gut feeling" is probably most important. If you think that your child is really sick, call your doctor and ask to be seen immediately. If your doctor is not available or cannot see your child promptly, rush to the nearest emergency room and request that your child be seen immediately.

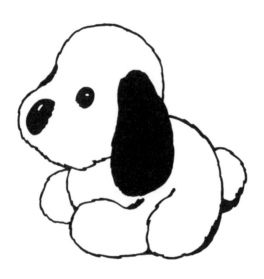

Seven

Caring for Your New Infant

Holding your new baby

A new baby's muscles are not strong enough to support his or her head until around three months of age. It is important to remember this when you hold or carry your baby. You can support your child's head easily in the crook of your arm. If you hold the baby upright against your chest, or with the head resting on your shoulder, be sure to support the head with your hand.

When to feed your baby

Feed your baby whenever he or she is hungry. Do not put your baby on a schedule. After a few months, baby will set his or her own schedule.

You can start your baby on low-fat (2 percent) or homogenized milk at nine to twelve months of age. Feed your baby the milk you use, cold out of the refrigerator, and make the baby a member of the family. All babies need some fat to grow; do not use nonfat milk.

True milk allergy is uncommon, but milk intolerance is common. If your baby does not do well on a milk formula, changing to a soy formula may help.

Your baby's appetite will probably decrease during the hot summer months. However, fluids are important and should be encouraged. Remember, your baby will eat and drink what he or she needs if you make it available.

What to feed your baby

Nutritionally your baby does not need anything except breast milk or formula until six months of age. If you like you can offer your infant some water in between feedings. Most babies do not like water and refuse it. If that happens, do not worry, both breast milk and formula contain plenty of free water to take care of the baby's needs. Some time after three weeks of age, solids such as baby rice cereal given late in the evening may make your baby sleep longer.

Bottles

There are few real pleasures in life, and, to a baby, having a bottle is one of them. The important point is not for your baby to give up the bottle, but to learn to drink from a cup. Once your baby learns this, around nine months of age, a few bottles a day are not a problem.

There is no specific age when you have to stop the bottle. After two years of age bottles are not appropriate in public, but are OK at home (nap-, sad- and bedtime).

Bottles with sugar-containing fluids such as

milk and juice must be finished promptly and *not* be sipped on. Children who continually sip on bottles with milk or sugar-containing fluids get tooth decay we call bottle caries. This destroys their front teeth.

If your baby needs to carry a bottle and sip occasionally for security, give him or her a plain water bottle. This will not hurt the teeth.

Pacifiers

Most children like to suck. It gives them security.

Pacifiers are wonderful: They give *parents* many hours of peace and quiet.

Pacifiers all work the same, use one that your baby likes. They do not deform the teeth or cause your child to need braces in the future.

If you don't offer a pacifier, your baby may

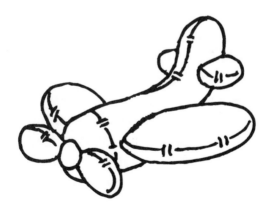

start sucking his or her thumb. Thumbs do push on the palate and teeth, which may result in the need for braces in the future. Offer a pacifier early, so that your baby does not start sucking on his or her thumb. Thumbs are firmly attached and cannot, eventually, be thrown away.

Security blankets

Security blankets are common.

They make your child feel good and are harmless.

Clean the security blanket occasionally. It eventually falls apart and is gone.

Best Advice:

Do not worry, nobody goes to high school with a bottle, pacifier or security blanket.

Vitamins and fluoride

Babies need vitamins to grow and develop normally. Most babies do get enough vitamins from their formula and the solid foods they eat. To make sure that the baby does get enough vitamins, most doctors recommend supplementary vitamin drops to be started between one and four months of age. This is reassurance that the baby gets all the "goodies" needed to grow on.

Fluoride is important to strengthen the baby's teeth and works well to prevent future decay and cavities. The baby's permanent teeth start forming shortly after birth and are made up of calcium. Fluoride supplement can be given either combined with vitamins or separately.

The fluoride is utilized as "building blocks" for the teeth as they are formed and will be there permanently.

This is different from the fluoride treatment which the dentist will later paint on your child's teeth. Fluoride applied to the outside coats the teeth and protects them, but is not incorporated into the actual structure of the tooth. It is like a brick facing for a house, rather than having a house built of brick.

Some communities fluoridate their drinking water. That works well if the baby drinks enough water.

For most busy parents, the vitamin fluoride combinations work best. Ask your doctor to recommend one.

Best Advice:

Make sure your doctor prescribes vitamins with fluoride in the first few months after birth.

House temperature

Keep the temperature in your home the way you like it.

Dress your baby in the same amount of clothes that you need to keep comfortable.

Washing your baby

Wash or bathe your baby daily and whenever he or she is dirty. You can use any of the many special baby soaps available at the drugstore. However, your baby does not need a special soap and does well with whatever soap you already have for yourself at the sink or in the tub. Sponge-bathe your baby until the umbilical cord has fallen off. Use a water temperature that is comfortable to you; it will be comfortable for baby as well.

If your baby has dry skin, bathe him or her only every other day. Wash dirty areas as necessary.

For dry or sensitive skin you can use Aveeno or Neutrogena soap.

Never, ever leave a baby in a bath alone, not even for one second.

After baby's bath:

Baby oil may make your baby slippery.

Powders are fine if you like them.

Baby-lotion makes your baby smell good.

Washing your baby's clothes

Wash your baby's clothes in the same detergent you use for your regular laundry.

Bottom care

Your baby's bottom needs regular cleaning. Keep an unbreakable plant-misting bottle where you change diapers and spray the baby's bottom when it is dirty; it makes it easier to clean. Change the water in the spray bottle daily.

Calming your baby

You can't spoil your baby in the first few months of life.

If your baby cries, check to see if he or she is hungry or dirty. If the crying continues, pick up your baby and comfort him or her. This will usually make your baby happy.

What if your baby is fussy or screaming, but has been fed and diapered, and you have tried everything, yet nothing seems to help? Remember, sometimes babies just cry, for no good reason. This is normal.

Don't try to calm your baby by jiggling, bouncing from shoulder to shoulder, or other strenuous activity. All this just stimulates and stresses the baby's nervous system and often causes more wailing. Instead place your baby in one spot, tummy down on a flat surface or across your knees, gently stroke the back, and talk or croon in a steady, calm voice. A little rocking may help, as does sucking on a pacifier (the baby, not you).

Parents often feel they have to do something when their baby fusses, but most of the time babies will settle down by themselves after a little while, so relax and wait it out. (Well, try.)

Cigarette smoke

Babies who live in homes where there is cigarette, cigar or pipe smoke have more upper respiratory tract infections, ear infections and asthma. Do not smoke or allow others to smoke around your baby.

Shyness and babies

Around nine to fifteen months of age, most babies become very suspicious of strangers. This usually lasts until about three years of age. The best way to handle this is to not force someone new on the child, but wait for the toddler to come to this person when he or she is ready to make friends.

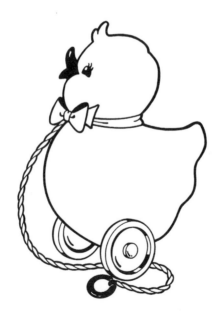

Eight

Common Health Concerns—Infants

Baby acne

Many babies get a red, bumpy rash over their face, forehead and scalp. This is called baby acne. It disappears around seven to nine weeks of age. If it bothers you, a little Cortaid (.5 percent cortisone) rubbed on several times a day will make it fade sooner.

Baby jaundice

One out of every two babies gets a little yellow or jaundiced between two and six days of age. This is more common in breast-fed babies.

Give your baby extra water, and place baby by the window into diffuse sunlight (not into direct sunlight or the baby will sunburn). If your baby is acting and eating OK and is not dark yellow, do not worry. The jaundice will clear up in a few days.

Birthmarks

Birthmarks are common in babies. Most of these will fade with time, but a few will remain and may even grow.

Almost all infants have several pale pink-red marks called nevus flammeus. They are usually on the forehead, eyelids and the back of the head near the neck. They also are called stork-bite marks and almost always fade and disappear.

A similar mark which is a darker red is called a port wine stain. These birthmarks may be fairly large and can be anywhere on the body. They are permanent and do not go away. If the mark is on the forehead or near the eyes your doctor should consider a serious condition called Sturge-Weber, which may include seizures, glaucoma and developmental delay.

Dark blue marks which look like bruises are called Mongolian spots. They are more frequent in Oriental infants and dark-skinned babies. They are commonly found over the buttocks, but can be up and down the back and the shoulders. These birthmarks are harmless and also fade somewhat. It is important to realize that Mongolian spots are not bruises and the child has not been injured.

Moles normally appear as the child gets older. Some babies are born with moles. These may be small or quite large and some have hairs growing out of them. Moles present at birth are called congenital moles and should be watched by the doctor, especially if they are large. Congenital dark brown moles are more likely to turn malignant and the larger ones should be removed before or at puberty.

A very common birthmark is the capillary hemangioma or strawberry birthmark. These may be present at birth or appear over the first few months of life.

The strawberry birthmark starts as a small, bright red spot which rapidly grows up and out, and really does look like a strawberry. It may grow to be quite large and there may be many of them over the body. This birthmark always goes away during the first five years of life and leaves no scars. If treated, scars almost always form.

Unless the birthmark blocks an eye and prevents vision, which would put the baby at risk of a blind eye (amblyopia ex anopsia; see cross-eyes, page 40) or the birthmark ulcerates and bleeds or becomes seriously infected, no treatment is indicated.

Light brown birthmarks with irregular borders are quite common. They may be quite large, but are usually not unsightly and there is no treatment. Light brown birthmarks which have round, smooth borders are called *"cafe au lait spots"* (coffee and cream). If there are many it may mean that the child has a potentially serious condition called neurofibromatosis that you doctor can diagnose and discuss with you.

Best Advice:

Birthmarks are common and usually cause no problem. Most go away without treatment. If you are worried, ask your doctor if you should see a skin specialist.

Blocked tear-ducts

A blocked tear-duct in one or both eyes is common at birth. The baby's eye or eyes drain clear fluid, the lubrication tears, out of the corners. This occurs because the drainage into the nose is partially blocked. Most of these blocked tear-ducts open by themselves before the baby is a year old.

Rinse eyes out using a cotton ball dipped in saltwater (one cup water into which you put 1/4 teaspoon salt; bring this mixture to a boil and then cool). Dunk the cotton in the sterile saltwater and gently move it over the infant's closed eyes. Enough will go into the eyes to rinse them out. Take your child to your doctor or an eye specialist if the eyes still drain at one year of age or at any time if the eyes become red or swollen.

Bowel movements

How often the baby "goes to the bathroom" is very important to most parents. It is not very important to most babies.

Each baby is different. Some go often, some go only every few days. There is no right or wrong schedule.

Immediately after your baby is born, the color of the stool is dark green. When your baby is a few days old, the stool turns to a bright yellow or orange color.

The stool may be hard, soft or watery. Many

babies groan, grunt and get red in the face when they have a bowel movement. This is normal.

Breast lumps

Many new babies (boys and girls), especially those born a little early, have firm, movable lumps under each nipple during the first weeks of life. They may even leak a few drops of milk (witch's milk). This is normal and nothing to worry about. The lumps are caused by the mother's female sex hormone to which the baby is exposed while in the womb. These lumps are harmless and always go away during the first few weeks of life.

Some girl babies develop a little breast tissue late in the first year or early in the second year of life, and so have small breasts. This is called "premature thelarche." It may go away in a few months or persist. We do not know what causes it. As long as the baby is otherwise well, do not worry.

Constipation

A glycerin suppository inserted into the rectum (or the tip of your thermometer wiggled around a little) will make your baby have a bowel movement almost immediately.

Carnation Goodstart or Soyalac formula often makes the stools softer. Or you can mix:

1   teaspoon of dark Karo syrup
    (corn syrup)
1   ounce of water.

If your baby drinks this several times a day, the bowel movements will be more frequent and the stools looser.

If your baby is eating fruits, baby prunes will make the stools softer.

Several teaspoons of unmilled bran, mixed in cereal or applesauce, is healthy and makes stools softer and more frequent.

Best Advice:

Leave your baby alone. Having a bowel movement is something the baby will take care of all by itself.

Cephalhematoma

Some babies, after birth, develop a soft, fluid-filled "bump" over one or both sides of their head. This bump is caused by bleeding under the scalp. Cephalhematomas are harmless, painless and go away by themselves over several weeks. No treatment is necessary.

Colic

Nobody knows what causes colic. There are many theories, from gas pains to transferred parental stress.

Colic is more common in boys and firstborn children.

Your baby has colic if he or she cries inconsolably for several hours, usually in the evening. The legs are pulled up and the baby appears very uncomfortable. The stomach often rumbles and the baby passes lots of gas.

When not in pain, the baby is fine.

Babies with colic eat well.

Babies with colic grow well.

Babies with colic have normal bowel movements.

Babies with colic drive their parents crazy!

If you have never had a baby with colic, you cannot believe how stressful it is for everyone in the home.

Things to try:

- Breast-feeding mothers should stop drinking coffee, milk and cola-type (brown) soft drinks. They should stop eating milk products and chocolate. If this works, it works within forty-eight hours.

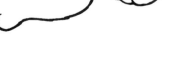

- If your baby is bottle-fed and is on a milk formula, you can try a soy formula.

- An over-the-counter "degasser," such as simethicone drops, occasionally gives relief.

- You can prepare good home remedies:

  A pinch of cumin.
  A pinch of oregano.
  Mix in 1-1/2 cups of water. Boil for 5 minutes. Strain the boiled mixture and add sugar to taste.
  Feed this warm to your baby as needed for colic.
  Or:
  1 yellow onion, cut up. Boil in 6 ounces of water until water is brownish. Cool, flavor with a little sugar. Feed 1-2 ounces warm to baby as necessary.

- Take your baby for a drive in the car, until the crying stops.

- Turn on a vacuum cleaner and place it touching the crib.

- Buy "Sleep Tight," a gizmo that simulates being driven in a car.

This is expensive, but works most
of the time. (You can later rent it to
friends and neighbors).

Best Advice:

*Do the best you can to keep your sanity.
Colic stops by itself around four months of age
and does not harm your baby.*

Cradle cap

Many babies get cradle cap. It is a form of
seborrheic dermatitis, similar to dandruff, and
often involves the scalp, part of the forehead and
face. With cradle cap, the scalp and skin are
dry. There is peeling, flaking and there may be
some redness.

Most parents do not like cradle cap and
worry, but there is no reason for concern. If your
baby has cradle cap it doesn't mean you aren't
a good parent. Here is what you can do: Wash
the baby's hair and face frequently. Or, you can
rub Cortaid (.5 percent cortisone) or Cortizone-
10 (1 percent cortisone) into the affected area
several times a day, then shampoo after two or
three days and the cradle cap will be gone.

Best Advice:

*Cradle cap is harmless. It does not mean
that you do not clean your baby. And even if
you do nothing, it eventually goes away .*

Cross-eyes (strabismus)

Cross-eyes is fairly common in children. For the first few months of life it is probably not important that the eyes line up. However, by four months of age your child's eyes must line up and look straight.

Pseudo-strabismus is when the eyes line up, but because of the folds along the inner eye and nose (called epicanthal folds) it looks as if the baby is cross-eyed when looking to either side. Your doctor can diagnose this and reassure you.

Strabismus can be caused by:

- Refractive error (nearsighted or farsighted).

- Imbalance of one or more of the six muscles that control each eyeball.

- Something serious inside the eye itself.

Remember that the muscles that control the eyes do get tired after prolonged use. If you notice that the child's eyes do not line up straight at home, ask your doctor to refer you to an ophthalmologist, even if in the morning, in the doctor's office, the eyes look perfectly straight.

This is what happens if your child's eyes do not line up perfectly: The back of the brain (the occipital cortex or vision area) receives two images (one from each eye) that are not superimposed. The human brain does not tolerate seeing things "double" and so it shuts off one image. The brain in that area, over time, loses the ability to function and that eye will become blind. This is called amblyopia ex anopsia and if not taken care of by age four will result in permanent blindness in the "off" eye!

Treatment may include:

- Glasses to correct any refractive error.

- "Patching" the good eye so that the bad eye must be used (and so stimulate the brain to function again).

- Eye-muscle surgery (or muscle-paralyzing medication injected into the tight muscle to lengthen it).

Best Advice:

Cross-eye must be diagnosed and corrected before four years of age. If your child's eyes look "crossed" to you, bring it to your doctor's attention and make sure that your child is sent for a competent eye evaluation. If your child's eyes were straight and suddenly cross, call your doctor immediately.

Diaper rash

You can cure most diaper rashes by keeping the diaper off and/or changing your baby more frequently. A good protective diaper ointment such as Balmex or Diaparene helps. If your usual diaper rash ointment does not cure the rash, it may be because the rash is caused by a fungal infection. Keep the diaper area clean, and blow-dry it with a hair-dryer on the "warm" setting (not "hot") after each diaper change. Try an antifungal cream such as Micatin or Lotrimin (miconazole or clotrimazole) that you can buy without a prescription.

Fleabite rash (erythema toxicum neonatorum)

Many babies have a spotty, red, bumpy rash, called a "fleabite" rash, all over their bodies in the first week of life. Do not worry; it has nothing to do with fleas and goes away by itself after a few days.

Heat rash

This rash is common during the hot weather. It looks like little red bumps. Keep your baby cool, in the shade, and use a bland powder on the skin. Clothing should be light and let air through.

Hernias

A hernia is an opening (hole) in the abdominal wall. Hernias are present at birth.

Hernias become noticeable when something, usually a loop of intestine, pokes through the opening causing a lump. This can happen at any age. Some hernias (umbilical) go away by themselves. In others (inguinal), you must close the opening or hole with surgery.

Umbilical hernias are present in all babies. The opening is the area where the umbilical cord entered the baby: the belly button.

. Umbilical hernias usually close by themselves over several months. Belly bands or coins taped over the belly button do not help.

An umbilical hernia that is still present at three years of age will probably not go away and will need surgical correction.

Inguinal hernias occur in the groin.

Inguinal hernias are more common in boys but do occur in girls.

During the baby's development an opening exists on each side of the groin so that in boys the testicle, which originates in the abdomen, has a pathway to travel into the scrotum (sack).

In girls the same pathway exists, though it is not used, as the ovary remains in the abdomen and does not travel down.

This opening usually closes before the baby is born. If it remains open, the baby has a hernia.

If a loop of intestine finds its way down through the opening, a lump appears in the groin. This lump may come and go, and is more prominent with crying or when the baby pushes to have a bowel movement.

When your baby relaxes, you can push it back up, only for it to reappear next time the baby cries.

An inguinal hernia does not go away. The only cure is surgical repair. As long as the hernia is present, there is the possibility that the loop of bowel will get trapped. This is an incarcerated inguinal hernia, and emergency surgery is necessary.

In little girls, occasionally, the ovary will herniate (come out) through the hole. There will be a tender lump in the lower abdominal area. Once out, the herniated ovary does not go back in and immediate surgery is necessary to save the ovary.

Best Advice:

If you think your child has an umbilical hernia, just watch it until your baby's next visit to the doctor, then point it out. If you think your child has an inguinal hernia, call your doctor.

Hydrocele (fluid around the testicle)

Around your boy's testicles is a thin membrane. This covers the testicle snugly like a glove. If fluid collects inside this membrane it balloons out, and the area on that side will appear large and swollen, a condition we call a hydrocele.

Hydroceles are common. They may be present at birth or show up in the first year of life. They can occur at any time after an injury to that area.

Hydroceles may be on one or both sides. They may be quite firm and large, but do not hurt or bother your baby.

Hydroceles are translucent. A light source (flashlight) placed behind the collection of fluid shines through it (which would not happen with a solid mass).

Babies with hydroceles also may have hernias.

Simple hydroceles often go away. A hydrocele still present at the end of the first year will probably not go away and should be removed surgically. Hydrocele surgery is a simple operation. If a hernia is present, the surgeon will fix that also.

We do not know what causes hydroceles. If your baby has one, watch it for at least the first year before you consider surgery.

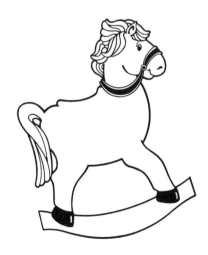

Infections

Babies do not handle infections well, especially in the first few months of life. Keep your baby away from crowds and, especially, from sick people.

Best Advice:

Any temperature above 100.8 degrees in a baby under three months of age is potentially dangerous! Call your doctor.

Spitting up
(esophageal reflux)

Many babies spit up a little, on and off. This is because the muscle at the opening of the stomach is loose, and some food runs back up. This is called esophageal reflux. Don't worry as long as your baby gains weight. If the frequent spitting up becomes a nuisance, this is what helps:

- Thicken the formula with some baby rice cereal (remember to make the nipple opening bigger).

- Don't bounce the baby around after a feeding, but hold him or her quiet and upright.

- When you do put the baby down, put him or her into an infant/car seat, in the upright position.

- Keep a burp rag between you and
  the baby to protect your clothes.

If the baby slowly loses weight, see your doctor. (See also Vomiting, page 48)

Teething

Teeth can come at any time between birth and eighteen months of age. They always eventually come!

You can help teething pain with baby Tylenol (acetaminophen). Cold teething rings also help.

Teething does *not* cause fever, but does lower baby's resistance to viral and other infections that may then cause some fever.

Thrush or monilia infection

Thrush, a monilia infection of the inside of the mouth, is common. Most babies have it at some time and it does not usually bother them. Monilia, a common fungus, lives inside the mouth, and when conditions are just right, enough of the fungus can grow to be visible as white, irregular patches which stick to the inner cheeks and gums. Thrush is often mistaken for milk which has adhered to gums and inner cheeks. Thrush can be treated with an oral medication (mycostatin), but even without treatment the white patches will go away by themselves. If the baby is breast-fed, an antifungal cream (Lotrimin or Micatin) can be used by the mother to prevent sore, cracked nipples.

Vaginal bleeding

Some little girls have some vaginal bleeding or mucus discharge from the vagina during the first week of life. This is caused by the mother's female sex hormone to which the baby was exposed in the womb. Do not worry; this is normal and it stops by itself.

Vomiting
(pyloric stenosis)

Real vomiting, where milk and food comes flying out, may happen during the first month or two.

If it persists, it may mean that the muscle at the far end of the stomach is too tight, so that the stomach cannot empty. This is called pyloric stenosis. The condition is more common in first-born boys and runs in families.

With pyloric stenosis, the vomiting gets progressively worse, and the baby loses weight. Pyloric stenosis has to be surgically corrected.

If your baby exhibits continued vomiting and/or weight loss, call your doctor.

(See also Spitting up, page 46)

Nine

Your Child's Development — the First Five Years

The years from one to five are turbulent and will try your patience. Our pleasant, friendly one-year-old becomes a completely different person, often changing back and forth from angel to monster.

Your baby and talking

During the first two years of life it is very important for your baby to develop listening and talking skills. Talking, singing and reading to your child will help him or her to learn to talk.

Three to four months: Baby listens when you talk. Sing and talk to your baby as much as possible in a pleasant voice. Worry if your baby does not seem to hear or listen to your voice.

Nine to ten months: Baby understands simple words like "no no." Baby indicates what he or she wants by pointing. Teach words by repeating them often (Mama, Da Da, bye-bye). Worry if your baby does not look at you when you talk to him or her.

Twelve months: Baby says one or two words. Points and babbles. Show your baby pictures and name objects in the environment. Worry if your baby does not point to things he or she wants.

Eighteen months: Baby says thirty or more words and follows simple directions. Teach songs, nursery rhymes and give simple commands for baby to follow. Worry if baby does not say more than five words.

Twenty months: Baby uses two-word sentences and follows simple directions, understands much of what you say and enjoys listening to you talking. Worry if your child does not follow simple commands like "Come to Mommy."

Two-plus years: Child likes listening to simple stories. Uses many words, putting several together. Worry if your two-year-old does not say fifty words or does not use two words together.

Best Advice:

Encourage baby to talk by talking and singing to him or her as much as you can. If your baby falls into the "worry" group, talk to your doctor for advice about what to do next.

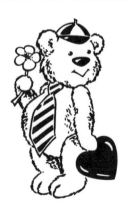

Here's what else to expect:

Eighteen months

The child is often negative. Everything is "No," but distraction is easy. Your child is mobile and gets around. Frustration often causes biting and hitting.

Two years

The child is calmer, but this age is only a breather to give Mom and Dad a momentary rest.

Two-and-a-half years

The child does not tolerate change in either the environment or daily routine. The toddler is easily upset, throws tantrums, is domineering and dictatorial. Choices only confuse and lead to wasted time. Mom and Dad must be positive, make decisions and avoid letting the child take charge.

Three years

This is a good time. "Yes" is more common, and instead of just taking, the child is ready to give and share a little. Rituals slowly disappear and people become more important. There may be a lot of crying and the child needs reassurance. Between three-and-a-half and four imaginary companions are common, particularly for only-children.

Four years

At this age, your child may often be out of bounds, defiant and boastful. Biting and hitting can occur with any frustration. Verbally there may be shouting and profanity. Lying is common.

Your four-year-old needs freedom to test the environment, but also needs firm limits and controls.

Five years

This usually is a good time. Your child is more secure, is agreeable, and loves Mom and Dad. Enjoy it!

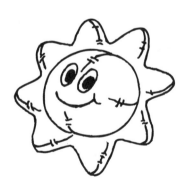

Ten

Caring for Your Toddler

Feeding your toddler

Toddlers like most foods and are willing to experiment with what is offered.

Feed your toddler your own food as much as possible and make him or her a member of the family. The three- to four-year-old does not need special foods.

Your child is growing fast. Meat and other proteins are important, as are fruits and vegetables. Offer these foods before you offer starches or dessert.

Milk and milk products supply the calcium necessary for bone growth. If your child does not like milk, the best and cheapest way to supply calcium is to give the child Tums. You can buy Tums at the drugstore. It comes in several flavors and is chewable. Two to three Tums daily will give your child all the calcium needed for good bone growth.

Give the child the meal you are serving but do *not* nag about eating. Meal times should be pleasant times. When eating stops, remove the food and send the child off to play. Do *not* feed your toddler between meals.

Most children do not eat as much as parents think they should. Remember, children are like little sports cars. When the gas tank is empty, they stop running. If your child is running around, feels well and seems happy, do not worry about the amount of food eaten. It is enough.

Best Advice:

Remember, you are not running a restaurant. Your toddler has to learn that food comes at meal times and that the only choice is to eat or go hungry.

Walking, feet and shoes

Most children walk when they are ready, between eight and eighteen months of age. Any time in this age-range is normal.

Most children, when they first stand and walk, point their feet either in, out or to the side for balance. Feet rarely point straight to the front at first.

The ankles roll inward, and the foot appears flat with little or no arch. This is due to loose ligaments and a little fat pad most babies have on their sole, filling the arch.

Many children look bowlegged.

This all corrects itself during the first few years without shoe-bars or expensive walking or orthopedic shoes. As your child gets older, the legs and feet will become straight.

Things to keep in mind about shoes:

- Shoes do not straighten feet or
  ankles.

- Shoes protect the foot from heat, cold and sharp objects.

- Shoes must be long enough and wide enough and the sole should be soft and flexible.

- High-top shoes are expensive and do nothing for feet or ankles. Tennis shoes are fine.

- Buy shoes that you like, that fit, that are soft and inexpensive—feet grow very fast.

Best Advice:

Your child will walk when he or she is ready. Your child's feet and legs will be OK if you leave them alone.

Bedtime

Toddlers thrive on routine and need a regular bed time.

Many toddlers are verbal and will try to bargain with you to stay up. Do not get into a discussion. Just say, "It's bedtime; let's go to bed," and put the child to bed.

If your child cries, return briefly to comfort him or her, but do not pick the child up.

If your toddler comes out of the bedroom repeatedly, restrain with a gate or other means (close the door). Do not feel guilty; children have *no* business wandering around the house at night.

Toddlers love to sleep in Mom's and Dad's bed during the night. Do not permit this! Every night your child spends in your bed will make it that much harder to get the child back into his or her own bed. Gate the child's bedroom door if necessary, leave a little night light on, and have bedtime, sleep-with toys available.

Best Advice:

Children and parents sleep better if all are in their own beds at night. Don't make a big to-do about bedtime. Be firm and consistent and you won't have much trouble.

Chronic loose bowel movements

There are few things as frustrating (and worrisome) to parents as the child who has one to four large, loose, watery bowel movements daily. This happens in children between nine months and two years of age. It frequently starts out with a mild upset stomach, with vomiting and diarrhea. The child gets better, eats well, but now has these really horrible stools.

The stool runs out of the diaper, is messy to clean up and drives everyone crazy! Parents often switch from doctor to doctor looking for a cure, but the awful stools continue for many months in spite of everything that is tried.

The best explanation for this pesky problem is that the bowel speed that pushes the digesting food along has increased and so less water (but not nutrients) is absorbed.

The most important thing is to realize that the child is *not* sick. Diarrhea is an illness: the child has lots of loose stools, does not feel well and is generally under the weather. Children with chronic loose stools *do* feel well, eat well, are gaining weight and are active.

What is a parent to do?

It is important for parents to remember that several loose, messy stools do not bother the child—just the parent.

You can try an over-the-counter product called Lactinex Granules (lactobacillus).

Sometimes giving the child a half teaspoon of cooking oil in food daily helps.

Best Advice:

If your child has many loose, messy bowel movements, but is growing well, eating well, is active and gaining weight, do not worry. Remain cheerful, clean up your child and wait it out. It usually gets better by itself.

Toilet training

You cannot make your child go to the bathroom.

If you push the child, your child realizes that

this is very important to you. It then becomes a game not to go. The child holds back, the stool dries out and becomes hard. When the child does go, it hurts. The pain makes the child hold back again, and a vicious circle starts: pain and holding. Now you have a real problem!

Children toilet train themselves when they are ready, usually somewhere between two and five years of age.

For toilet training, your child must have sensation, which comes first, and control, which usually comes six to nine months later.

Until this occurs, you cannot train the child.

Once children have sensation, they tell you when they are wet or dirty and want to be cleaned.

If you change the diaper or pull-up pants promptly, the time will come when you find your child is still clean. The child now can control or hold the bowel movement. From that time on, training rapidly takes place.

Night-training usually takes longer than day-training and many children still need diapers at night

If you use a potty chair for your child, keep it in your bathroom. When you go, take the child with you. Your child will play with the potty chair, and eventually will sit on it. Encourage, but do not push the child.

If you want your child to sit on the big toilet, turn the child around and let him or her hold on to the lid for support. You can stick a decal to the lid for your child to look at.

Best Advice:

All children toilet train themselves eventually. If you encourage and do not push the child, you won't have any problems.

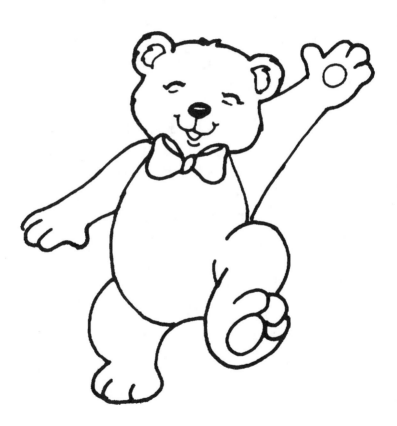

Playing with stool

Before your toddler is ready for toilet training, the sensation that something is happening occurs. This is a new feeling, and there is often much interest by the toddler in what is going on down there. Soon the child realizes that something has come out—has been produced. This is exciting! Often toddlers reach in their diaper to admire what is there, and then play with their stool, knead it or smear it around. This is fun for the baby, though not for the parents, who often despair and do not know what to do. Remember, this is not aberrant behavior; in fact this is common.

The child does not do it to spite the parents. The toddler is proud of what he or she has produced. The child does not consider the bowel movement dirty and so does not understand why parents get so upset. This is a phase that passes quickly.

Best Advice:

Clean your child and the environment, keep your sense of humor, and wait it out.

Biting

Between fifteen and twenty-four months of age, many toddlers will bite parents, siblings and any other child that is near when the toddler is frustrated or angry. This can be a real problem, especially if the child is in day care.

There is no good treatment for this. You must protect other children by removing your child for a brief time. This biting is normal behavior for the age and luckily does not last long. Children are very animalistic at this age and this is their way of showing their displeasure.

Best Advice:
If your child bites others, protect them and wait it out. It won't last long.

Water safety

Children most often drown in pools that are not fenced. These accidents usually happen in the family's, grandparents' or a neighbor's pool. The typical drowning victim is an active three-year-old boy who drowns in the family pool when left alone. The caretaker has left, just for a second, to answer the telephone, doorbell, or to get something from inside the house.

You cannot drown-proof a child. Fence your pool and get self-locking gates.

Infants and toddlers also frequently drown in the bathtub. Never leave your toddler unsu-

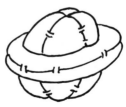

pervised during a bath, even if the phone or doorbell rings.

Learn CPR (cardiopulmonary resuscitation). Classes should be available from your local Red Cross chapter or at a local hospital. If you can get your child to breathe right after a drowning accident, your chances for a complete recovery are good.

Best Advice:

Never let your child out of your sight near water.

Pets

New pets and toddlers do not go well together. Puppies and kittens are never an appropriate gift for a toddler. Toddlers do not respect the animal's space and rights. They see kittens and puppies as inanimate objects similar to dolls that they can manhandle as desired.

If you have a dog or cat when the baby comes, the toddler and pet usually will get along. Not only will the pet be older, but the animal has seen the baby grow and become mobile. Older pets learn to avoid the rambunctious toddler and get safely out of the way.

Always keep your child away from an animal that is eating. Animals have little tolerance for children while they are eating and will bite to protect their food.

Always keep your child away from an animal with babies. A mother animal gets very protective and will bite if she thinks her little ones are in danger. Toddlers do not understand that animals are easily frightened and that animals will defend themselves by biting or scratching.

Best Advice:

No new puppy or kitten until your child is at least five years old.

Bed-wetting (enuresis)

Bed-wetting is a common problem in children, and often drives parents to distraction. Staying dry at night is developmental, and may happen any time between eighteen months and several years of age.

Remember:

- Children toilet train themselves when they are ready, usually between two and five years of age. Before that, most of them cannot stay dry. Do not get into a power struggle by trying the impossible.

- Emotional problems infrequently cause bed-wetting.

- Your child does not want to wet and is as unhappy about it as you are.

- Bed-wetting is more common in

boys, and there is often a family history of it.

- If your child is developmentally not ready, you cannot train him or her.

- If the child is ready, training will happen with little encouragement.

- The more you push the child, the less likely he or she will stop.

Some things to try after your child is six years old or older:

- There are several "wake-up" or conditioning devices on the market. With most a bell rings with the first few drops of urine to wake the child. This teaches the child to wake up and go to the bathroom. These devices work well, if your child is not a heavy sleeper.

- Antispasmodic medication, especially Ditropan, works occasionally, but probably not enough to make it your first endeavor at solving this problem.

- The best way to treat bed-wetting is with DDAVP or desmopressin acetate. DDAVP is similar to antidiuretic hormone which our body makes to regulate how often we urinate. Antidiuretic hormone is found in lesser amounts in bed-wetters. DDAVP is artificially made and comes in a squirt bottle as a nasal spray, given at bedtime. It works well, but you will need a pre-scription to get it. It is expensive and is most effective after six years of age.

Antidepressant medications work in some children. We do not know how they work; they just do. They may be used to allow an older child to spend sleep-overs with friends or be dry at camp. As these drugs are potentially danger-ous, you should not use them without close su-pervision by your doctor.

Best Advice:

Don't get discouraged. Almost all children will eventually be dry at night.

Communicating respect and values

Listen to your child. Talk to, not at, your child. Be quick to praise, and don't always instruct or complain.

However, don't overindulge your child. You must learn to distinguish between the child's needs and wants. You must teach your child to respect the rights of others, including your rights as a parent. Your child's wants should come after your needs and only as time is available.

Working parents have limited time, and children do not need, nor should they get, every free moment.

Many working parents feel guilty for leaving their children during the day. They try to make it up by indulging the child when they come home in the evening. This is wrong and does not help the child to grow up. All parents need time for themselves and occasional time away from their children. Children must get used to this separation and become used to others, such as baby-sitters. Children must learn to play alone and to wait.

Don't always rescue your child from everyday frustrations. Your child must learn how to cope. Be available and supportive and provide comfort when your child fails or is frightened.

Traveling

Traveling with children is never easy. If traveling with your child is hard for you, remember it is equally hard (if not harder) for the child.

It will take some planning before and during the trip to make it all tolerable for everyone. If you plan well, and everyone keeps the right attitude, traveling may even prove to be fun.

Car trips: Children quickly get bored, hungry and have the need to go to the bathroom. Prepare for this by taking along plenty of toys, reading material, games, food and drink. Plan on frequent (at least every one and a half to two hours) pit-stops to use the toilet and to let the child run off some of the accumulated energy. With older children play games such as looking for special license plates, road signs or animals along the highway. Always be sure everyone stays buckled in.

Airplane rides: Small children do not like being in a plane after the excitement of taking off and being in the air has lost its thrill. Airplane rules are strict and the child must remain seated and belted in most of the time. This is pure misery for the active toddler who wants to be up and going in this new and fascinating place.

Most sedatives given by a doctor to calm the child do not work because of the initial noise and excitement.

Don't plan on peace and quiet. Make the best of it, keep the child restrained and as happy as possible and focus on the fact that it will be over before long.

Once you have arrived at your destination, remember that it will be a strange often scary place full of strangers for the smaller child. Toddlers become grumpy or clingy and drive you and everyone crazy. Be patient and understanding. Let them become familiar with the new surroundings and people slowly.

Plan some fun things for the small child. Local playgrounds, the zoo, and, of course, toy stores are great.

These expeditions are good cultural experiences, and necessary for growing up. This lets children know that you have thought of and considered their interests, and that the trip is not only for you but also for them.

Day care

If Mom and Dad both have to work and no close relative is available, day care may be the answer.

Check your neighborhood for what is available and personally look at any place where you consider leaving your child.

What to look for:

- Is the day care's license up to date?

- How many children are usually there?

- Who and how many people take care of the children?

- What age children are there besides your child?

- Is the children's area neat and clean?

- What is the day care's policy if a child is ill?

- Is your child fed and changed as needed?

- What is the policy if your child gets sick while at day care?

- What is the policy if you are occasionally late picking up your child?

- Does the staff have a similar philosophy to yours on child care?

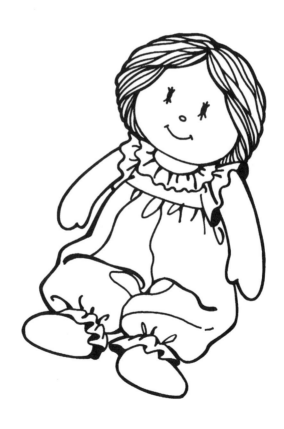

- Is the day care easy to get to, and the cost reasonable?

What to expect:
- In day care your child will be on a different routine than at home. This will not hurt the child.

- In day care your child will be with other children and so exposed to new viruses and bacteria. The number of colds, coughs, ear infections, and bouts of diarrhea will increase. Remember that this is how your baby develops immunity. There will be fewer infections later in childhood.

Best Advice:

Day care is a compromise. Nobody will look after your child exactly the way you do. You are looking for good, basic child care and peace of mind while you work. Day care can be a good experience for both child and parent.

Jealousy with a new brother or sister

When a new baby comes your other children will be jealous. Even little ones can sense that something is happening.

Jealousy is instinctive and always occurs.

Your children will feel just as Mom would feel if Dad brought a girlfriend home. Mom would probably move out, but your little ones cannot.

Children know that when you get something new, you often throw the old one away. Often they try hard to suppress any anger or jealousy that they feel. They want to be good, so that you do not throw them away.

There may be new behavior patterns. These often include:

- Direct physical or verbal attacks on the baby.

- Over concern and affection for the baby.

- Change in sleeping, in eating, in toilet habits, or an increase in attention-getting, obnoxious behavior.

It helps to include your children, starting with the pregnancy.

- Make your children feel wanted and helpful by letting them participate in care for the baby, with praise and reward for a job well done.

- Try to spend some extra time with the older children when the baby is sleeping.

• Make sure that visitors not only praise the baby but also the older children.

Best Advice:

Be patient. Older children slowly become used to the new arrival. Help them by making it everyone's baby.

Dreams, nightmares and night terrors

Dreams are common in babies, toddlers and older children. They often roll, thrash, and groan or make noises during their sleep as the events of the day are relived.

After four years of age real nightmares may occur. The child is afraid, cries out while sleeping and may actually panic and be inconsolable. Often there is sleepwalking. With minimal effort the child will wake up, may or may not remember the dream, and after settling down will go peacefully back to sleep. An occasional occurrence like this is not serious and probably does not warrant a visit to the doctor.

Night terrors differ from nightmares. The child is deeply asleep, but looks and acts as if awake and disoriented. The eyes may be wide open, parents are not recognized, and there may be random screaming, talking, walking or running around. This is really frightening for parents.

There is no good treatment; the child must

be fully awakened to stop the night terror. This is best accomplished by taking the child to the bathroom (well lighted) and washing his or her face with cool water. Usually after a few minutes the child wakes up, fusses a while and then goes back to sleep. There is usually no memory of the event.

Night terrors and nightmares will not harm your child. However, if they occur frequently they disrupt the whole house, and you should check with your doctor to discuss trying a brief course of medication to stop them.

Poison control

Around seven to nine months of age, your child becomes mobile and you must poison proof your home.

This includes:

- Keep the telephone numbers of your doctor and the local poison control center where you or your baby-sitters can immediately find them.

- Put safety latches on all closets and cupboards containing clean-ing materials and other household supplies.

- Put medicines safely away, prefer-ably under lock and key. Toddlers climb, so just putting them on a high shelf or counter is not enough.

- Parents, grandparents and other visitors must never leave purses where a toddler can get into them.

- Never put anything poisonous into a soft-drink bottle or other container that normally contains food products.

- Buy a one-ounce bottle of syrup of ipecac and have it available in your home. If your child eats or drinks a poison, this medication will cause vomiting. Never use syrup of ipecac without first checking with your doctor or the local poison control center!

Best Advice:

Poison prevention takes continual vigilance and work. Prevention is better than cure.

Lead exposure

Lead exposure has become an important environmental health issue. While there is little question that lead in large doses is dangerous, there is no consensus as to how dangerous minute lead levels really are. Recent reports, however, indicate that even very low blood lead levels may be harmful to the brains of growing children.

The potential sources of lead are:

- Lead-based paint. Any home built before 1980 is a possible source of lead-based paint.

- Dust and/or soil contaminated with lead from lead-based paint or leaded gasoline.

- Some folk remedies from Third World countries used for teething may contain lead. Do not use any medication for teething that was made in a foreign country.

- Food (usually imported) in lead-soldered cans.

- Imported decorated dishes or handmade pottery. Do not use pottery to prepare, cook or store food or drinks.

- Parents who work at jobs with lead exposure may bring it home on their clothes.

Children who are at risk include toddlers living in older homes, because they may chew on painted furniture or window sills; children going through a prolonged phase where they eat dirt outside, in the street, or back yard (interestingly, this is called pica, the Latin word for magpie, a bird which will eat anything); and children whose parents work in a lead-contaminated environment.

It is important to prevent lead exposure in all children.

A reasonable approach is:

- Check for potential lead exposure in your child's environment and, if found, take steps to eliminate it.

- If you are uncertain if your child has been exposed to lead, work with your doctor to develop a history for possible exposure.

- Laboratory screening is called for in children at risk by history.

Best Advice:

You will hear a lot about lead from friends, neighbors and the newspaper. Selective lead testing in children at risk of exposure is important, but universal lead screening is probably not necessary.

If you have questions, ask your doctor.

Eleven

Discipline

A child who isn't taught, early in life, that there are limits to acceptable behavior becomes an unhappy, unpleasant youngster and stands an excellent chance of becoming a frustrated, unhappy—perhaps even criminal—adult.

All children misbehave occasionally. As parents, it is our job to correct unacceptable behavior so that it does not reoccur.

A consistent show of disapproval for bad behavior must start no later than nine months of age. Begin with simple rules: Staying in the car seat, not biting or hitting others, going to bed. Enforce these and do *not* negotiate. Expect some crying but do not allow temper tantrums.

Be persistent and do not feel guilty. An occasional "no" is good; your child will still love you. You do not want a spoiled, undisciplined child who is manipulative and unpleasant.

Best Advice:

You cannot run your house like a democracy. Run your home as a benign dictatorship. This will help to make your home happy and peaceful and will make your child feel loved and secure.

Punishment

Punishment is one of the tools (along with verbal guidance and setting a good example) we use to teach a child about right and wrong. The child learns by experience that improper behavior results in something unpleasant happening to the child. To avoid this, the child—we hope—gives up the unacceptable behavior.

To be effective, punishment must possess two characteristics. It must be immediate (especially with younger children), and it must be disagreeable to the child.

Punishment also must be consistent over time. Don't punish a particular behavior and then later, under the same circumstances, allow it. This simply confuses the child and, in many instances, is worse than no punishment because the child will continue to push the limits in an attempt to discover what is permissible.

Punishment that is acceptable or appropriate at one age may not be acceptable or appropriate at another age. With young children there are two basic types of punishment:

- Corporal punishment: This includes spanking and light tapping. This startles the child, gets his or her attention, and creates some bodily pain which the child finds unpleasant.

- Time out: This consists of isolating the child for some time and withdrawing attention (and by implication, love) from the child. The child is confined to his or her room, has to stand in a corner, or in other ways is restricted for a period of time.

There is much controversy over what is the best way to punish a child. Some believe even minimal spanking is child abuse, teaches the child to use violence to solve problems, and is an infringement of the child's rights. However,

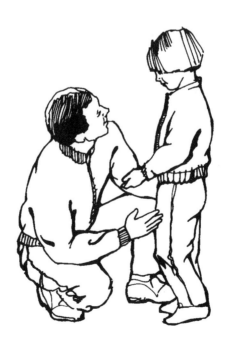

the American Academy of Pediatrics, the main child advocate in America, now believes that some spanking may be appropriate to change behavior. It goes without saying, of course, that no child should ever be beaten.

What is a parent to do? Here are some reasonable guidelines:

- Under nine months of age any form of punishment is inappropriate. The child is not old enough to understand and learn. Simply remove and distract the child from what he or she is doing.

- After nine months, raising your voice, frowning and chiding the child will be effective for a period of time.

- By 15 months, a firm "no" and maybe a slap on the child's diapered bottom or light tap on the fingers will startle the child, show your disapproval, and have the desired effect.

- From three to five years, time out may be productive. An occasional tap on the bottom will have the desired result and may be more effective. At this age you can begin to reason with your child. Explain why the particular behavior is unacceptable.

- Six years of age into the early teens can be a difficult time. If you have been loving yet firm with your discipline in the preceding years, these trying years should be easier. Time out and, with the younger child, an occasional spank are things to try. Withdrawal of privileges is often effective. Continue to explain to the child the reason his or her behavior is inappropriate. Be sure to be consistent.

- With the teen years, reasoning should be your main tool for behavior control. Back this up, however, with firm rules that, when violated, result in withdrawal of privileges. Limiting your child's use of the telephone or the car or complete grounding for a time period are usually effective. The teenager with firm rules to obey and the knowledge that consistent, fair punishment follows infractions is much more secure and happy than the unrestricted teen.

If you find you are having trouble disciplining your child, check with your doctor or with school administrators for adult classes, family counseling, local community groups, or other available resources that offer parental support in this important responsibility.

Best Advice:

Punishment must be swift, consistent, fair, memorable and used judiciously.

Twelve

Common Health Concerns—Toddlers

Baby measles (roseola infantum)

Roseola (a viral illness) is a common cause for fever in the first two years of life. It is rare before three months of age and usually does not occur after four years.

This disease is caused by human herpes virus 6 (HHV6), a common virus. The baby suddenly gets a very high fever (103°-105° F) with few if any other symptoms.

After three to seven days the fever suddenly drops and a spotty red rash appears which lasts for a few hours or days. As the rash appears, the fever ends and the child becomes very cranky for one or two days. The diagnosis cannot be made until the typical rash comes. Treatment consists of fever control with Tylenol (acetaminophen) or liquid Advil or Motrin (ibuprofen) available at the drugstore.

Fever convulsions may occur with roseola. They are very scary but are not harmful to your child. (See also Fever convulsions, page 89)

Best Advice:
Always call your doctor when your child has a high fever.

Choking

Choking is common in children. Choking deaths are most common in children five years or younger, and over half are in infants under two years of age. The most common causes are round food items such as grapes, pieces of hot dog, and candy. Small rubber toys, balloons, earrings, and other debris that the child finds on the floor also are dangerous.

All of these, on their way into the lung, block the air passages and can cause death if not removed. If your child aspirates something and is breathing, coughing or talking do not do anything. The chances are good that the child will cough out the obstructing object. If the child cannot make sounds, breathe and is turning blue, urgent help is needed. Do not try to fish anything out of the mouth that you cannot actually see. Lifting the lower jaw and tongue may help to let some air in. Call 911 for help.

A specific treatment for choking called the Heimlich maneuver helps to save lives. Check with your local Red Cross, American Heart Association, or if there is one nearby, a children's hospital, for a course that teaches you how to do this maneuver.

Best Advice:

Prevention is best. Be careful what you feed your child and with what toys your child plays.

Croup

This is a viral illness common during the winter and spring months. This disease is the same as laryngitis in adults.

Croup occurs in children between one and three years of age. The child starts with a little cold, and then wakes up at night with a seal-like or barky cough. Often there is real difficulty breathing in. (In asthma the difficulty is in breathing out).

Steam often gives relief. If you do not have a humidifier or vaporizer, the shower turned on to hot will make enough steam to help. A good expectorant cough medicine is often useful. Fever, if present, is low-grade (101°-102° F). Most children will improve as daylight comes, only to get sick again the next night or two.

A prescription steroid (cortisone-like) medication given by mouth helps after several hours, so it must be given early in the day to work that night. If breathing difficulty is severe, an inhalation treatment at the emergency room or even hospitalization may be necessary.

(See also Epiglottitis, page 88; and Asthma, page 128)

Ear infections (otitis media)

You may wonder: Why does my child get all those ear infections (and why can't my doctor do something to stop them)?

Over 75 percent of all children will have at least one ear infection before the age of three years. Most children will have many ear infections in the first two years of life.

This is what is known about this common nuisance:

- Age: Children who have their first ear infection during the first year of life usually have many more in the following two years.

- Environment: Household smoking irritates the membranes of the nose and throat. This makes children more susceptible to respiratory tract infections (colds) and thus to ear infections.

- Breast-feeding: This transfers some immunity which helps to protect the child.

- Bottle-feeding: If the baby is bottle-fed while lying down, there is more chance of infected secretions being forced up into the ears through the Eustachian tubes which connect the middle ear to the back of the throat.

- Day care: The child is exposed to more viral and bacterial infections of the respiratory tract, increasing the number of ear infections. Respiratory viruses alter the body's defense mechanism and make it easier for bacteria to grow. (Bacteria seem to be involved in about 75 percent of ear infections).

The pain can be treated with baby Tylenol (acetaminophen) or a similar medication or a combination of antibiotics and Tylenol. Keep the child's head and chest propped up at twenty to thirty degrees. Put a few drops of warm mineral oil into the infected ear every few hours. Salt water nose drops (one cup water, 1/4 teaspoon salt) help clear the nose.

Antibiotics do usually help, but even without them the earache will go away and the ear will heal by itself most of the time. The antibiotic amoxicillin is inexpensive and the drug of choice, but there are many others that can be used. Failure of antibiotic treatment is usually due to a viral infection (viruses are unaffected by antibiotics) present at the same time in the middle ear.

Recurrence after a course of antibiotic treatment is common. Eighty percent of recurrences are due to a new ear infection and not due to antibiotic failure. Ninety-five percent of all cases of otitis media are free of bacteria within five days of starting antibiotics.

Fluid will remain in the middle ear after an infection for two to sixteen weeks or even longer.

This may temporarily decrease your child's hearing a little but is not cause for alarm. Only if the fluid persists for six months or longer or there is escalated hearing loss do you have to worry.

Prophylactic (low dose) antibiotics daily for several months are effective in preventing recurrent ear disease. Your doctor should try this before the placement of tympanostomy tubes (tubes surgically inserted into the middle ear for drainage) is considered.

Best Advice:

Ear infections are common, and probably not avoidable. Treatment with simple antibiotics and Tylenol gives rapid relief and cures most of them. Tympanostomy (ear draining) tubes are the last resort.

Epiglottitis

Epiglottitis starts with croup-like symptoms, but the child rapidly becomes very ill. There is a high fever (103°-104° F), very sore throat and drooling. The cough is muffled, the child has real difficulty breathing in and sits up, with the head thrust forward for more air.

This is a life-threatening illness. Call your doctor immediately!

(See also Croup, page 85; and Asthma, page 128)

Fever convulsions

Fever convulsions are common in children six months to three years of age. They occur most frequently from six to eighteen months, and are very rare after four years of age.

They frighten parents, and parents feel helpless because they do not know what to do.

Fever convulsions are short and stop by themselves. Fever convulsions do not cause brain damage or death. Fever convulsions do not cause epilepsy later in life.

About six out of a hundred children will have one or more fever convulsions. Fever convulsions are caused by a high fever, but the child usually has only a simple viral illness. The rapid climb of the fever is what causes the seizure. The most important way to prevent a fever convulsion is to keep your child's fever down.

Take the child's temperature every three hours so you know what it is. Use Tylenol (acetaminophen) or similar products such as Advil or Motrin (ibuprofen) liberally when your child has a high fever.

If your child has a fever convulsion, put the child on his or her side. This helps any mucus or other matter in the mouth to come out, rather than being sucked into the lungs.

Call your doctor, but by the time you reach him or her, the convulsion probably will be finished. Follow your doctor's directions about what to do.

Common Myths:

- The child may die during a fever convulsion. This is not true. Simple fever convulsions are harmless.

- The child will be brain-damaged from the convulsions. This is not true. Fever convulsions do not cause brain damage.

- The child will get epilepsy later on. This is not true. Fever convulsions do not cause epilepsy. However, children who will get epilepsy later on also can have fever convulsions.

(See also Fever, page 142)

Best Advice:

If your child develops a fever, try to keep it below 102 degrees. If a convulsion occurs, keep calm, do not panic. Call your doctor. Your little one will be all right. If your child looks ill, regardless of what the fever is, call your doctor.

Head lice

Scalp infections with head lice are common during the preschool and school years. Children are very sociable and like to share hats, combs, ribbons and clothing with their friends. To prevent lice, teach your child not to borrow or use someone else's ribbons, scarves, towels, brushes, hats or combs.

If your child's scalp itches or is dry, look for lice and nits (louse eggs). You will find them behind the ears, at the crown and at the nape of the neck.

Carefully check the roots of individual hairs. Lice are tiny brown animals with many legs and they may move. They often cling to the roots of the hair. Nits are white, look like dandruff, but don't come out when you try to scrape them off.

You can buy several good medicated shampoos over the counter. Of the non-prescription drugs, Nix works best. Wash or dry-clean all clothes and bed linens. Seal unwashable items like stuffed toys in a plastic bag for ten days, or put them through the dryer on hot for a full cycle.

Best Advice:
Many children get lice. Do not feel ashamed. It does not mean you keep a dirty house. Just get rid of them.

Impetigo

Impetigo is a superficial skin infection that is very common in children and toddlers. It is almost always caused by a hemolytic streptococcus (the same bacterium that causes strep throat) or a staphylococcus, a bacterium that commonly lives on the skin and in the nose.

Impetigo can occur anywhere the skin breaks open (an injury, insect sting), but typically starts in the face around the nose, upper lip and mouth. Little red spots form which rapidly blister. The blisters break and form a thin, honey-colored crust. Several of these spots can join and the crusted area can become quite large. Impetigo is very contagious and can spread to any part of the body that the child touches and to other children and adults.

Treatment is with prescription antibiotics taken by mouth and with nonprescription antibiotic ointments (Neosporin, Polysporin) applied to the affected area after the crusts have been soaked off. A prescription ointment called Bactroban (mupirocin) applied three to four times a day to the crust works as well as oral antibiotics and your doctor may want to use this.

Best Advice:

Impetigo is a skin infection and is not caused by dirt. It is very contagious, so make sure that everyone's hands are washed thoroughly. Call your doctor for treatment with antibiotics by mouth or local application. This rapidly cures your child.

Infectious mononucleosis

This is a viral disease sometimes called the "kissing disease" or simply "mono." It is common in children of all ages. It is mildly contagious, spread by close contact but not necessarily by kissing.

Basic hygiene (hand washing, no mouth kissing) is adequate. Vigorous attempts to protect the other family members are not necessary. Mono is not that contagious. The chances are very good that the rest of the family will not get it.

Mono starts with a sore throat and swollen glands in the neck. Eventually the glands in the armpits and groin become large and swollen. After a few days the throat is covered with a thick film of whitish pus. Older children, especially teenagers, become very tired and want to sleep all the time.

Many teenagers are completely incapacitated by this disease. At the onset it is difficult to differentiate mono from a streptococcal sore throat. Any sore throat which does not improve in a few days, especially after antibiotics are started, is mono until proven otherwise. A blood count and a mono spot test (this test turns positive after several days if the disease is present) help make the diagnosis.

If your child has mono the only treatment is rest, a good diet and a daily multivitamin. It usually takes two weeks for the child to improve and then another two to three weeks before the child is cured. As the mono test remains positive for a long time, it does not help in pinpointing the end of the disease. After four to five weeks, if the child is better, the child can carefully return to regular activity.

Best Advice:

If your child has mono do not panic. He or she will improve and get better with rest.

Pinworms

Pinworms are very common in toddlers. They live in the lower part of the large intestine, and do not use any food or nutrients that your child needs.

Pinworms do not cause teeth grinding, convulsions or any other disease.

At night, during darkness, the female pinworm crawls out of the rectum to lay her eggs. This itches, causing the child to scratch. The eggs stick to fingers and hands, and in the morning are spread all over the house. Whatever the child touches will be covered with pinworm eggs. When these objects are handled, the eggs stick to fingers and hands. If the hands are not washed before the mouth is touched, the eggs are swallowed, and then hatch in the intestine causing new pinworms.

This cycle keeps repeating. If you have a toddler, your house, the preschool and all their friends' houses are covered with pinworm eggs, waiting to be swallowed.

Pinworms cause only three problems:

- If many worms come out of the rectum at night, the itching may be so intense that your child's bottom gets irritated. Then the discomfort and bottom-scratching will continue in the daytime.

- Mother or Father see the pinworms when changing the child's diaper and panic. Pinworms look like little pieces of white thread. The worms may be in the stool or around the rectum. This frightens parents.

- Sometimes, in little girls, a pinworm trying to crawl back into the rectum loses its way. It may then crawl into the vagina. This causes intense burning or itching. The little girl wakes up screaming and is inconsolable. To treat this: Place the little girl in a tub of warm water and let her soak until the worm drowns and she is comfortable. When the worm stops crawling, the pain and itching immediately go away.

If you think your child has pinworms, wait until around 11 p. m. and with a flashlight examine your child's rectum. Pinworms look like little white wiggly threads. If you find them, do not panic.

There is very effective prescription medication (Vermox) available. It is taken once and repeated a week later. This is not a cure; it just cuts down the number of worms and so improves the symptoms.

There is little use in treating family members who have no symptoms. As your environment is covered with pinworm eggs, everyone will immediately become reinfected.

As children get older, pinworms will disappear. Eventually children stop putting everything in their mouth, and they learn to wash their hands.

Best Advice:

In the long run pinworms are harmless. If you think your child has pinworms, call your doctor.

Scabies

Scabies are a little mite (insect-like creature) that burrows into the skin and then causes a rash which itches intensely. Your child gets scabies from close personal contact with someone who has scabies. Scabies is often found in several family members.

The mite burrows into the skin and forms a little tunnel where it lives. The entrance is often on the hands or feet. The tunnel is red and may look like an S-shaped line. The mite lays eggs, more mites hatch, crawl out, and burrow forming new tunnels.

Itching starts about a month after infection, as the child becomes sensitized to the mite. Itching is worse at night and scratching makes the rash worse. Infection often occurs in the scratched skin and this also changes the rash. Soon your child has an itchy rash all over, and looking at it one cannot readily tell what it is.

The diagnosis can be made by opening one of the tunnels and finding the mite or its droppings under the microscope. Often your doctor will presume that a rash is scabies and will treat it with medication. The best prescription medication is Elimite. This is painted on the skin and kills the mites.

As the mite dies in its burrow, the allergic reaction to its dead body gets worse, and often the rash and itching increase for several weeks. That does not mean the diagnosis was wrong or that the treatment did not work. The dead mite has to be absorbed before the child gets relief.

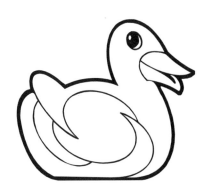

Treatment with a mild cortisone cream helps during this time. Other family members also should be treated at the same time. They are probably infected, even if not itching yet. Otherwise the scabies will spread again.

Best Advice:

Scabies comes from people who have scabies and is not caused because you keep a dirty house. If your child has a spreading rash that itches more at night, especially if other family members start itching or have a rash, think scabies. See your doctor for treatment and get rid of it.

Supermarket elbow
(subluxated radial head)

A pulled-out elbow is a common occurrence in babies and toddlers. Any sudden, sharp pull on the arm may pull out (subluxate) the radial head. (The radial head is the top of the radius, one of the lower arm bones, and it is supported only by a fibrous sling at the elbow.) Typically the child stands looking at something interesting in a store. The adult says, "Come, let's go," and pulls the child by the arm. Sometimes it happens when an adult picks the child up in fun by one or both arms to swing the child around. Sometimes the child just falls on the arm. The affected arm immediately hurts and the child will not use the lower arm, letting it hang down.

It is easy to pop the radial head back into place, an X-ray is not necessary and it does not have to be done immediately. When replaced, the pain is gone and the child again uses the arm. Call your doctor and ask what to do. Once an arm subluxates, it is more likely to happen again, and with less of a pull. If it occurs several times, ask your doctor to show you how you can put it back into place.

Best Advice:

Do not pick your child up by the arms, and be careful not to pull hard on the child's arms.

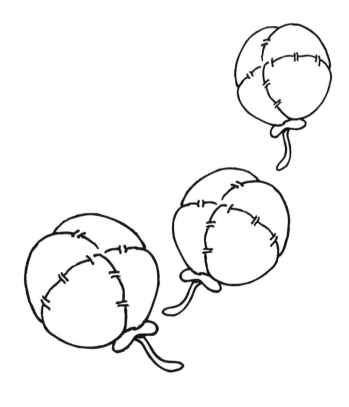

Tonsillitis
(sore throat, strep throat)

Tonsillitis is common in children and occurs all year long but is more common in the fall and winter. Most sore throats are caused by viruses and get better with pain relievers such as Tylenol (acetaminophen) and, for older children, gargling with hot water (salt is not necessary) several times a day. Antibiotics do not help and should not be used.

Streptococcal throat infections, or strep throat, is the only throat infection which *does* need antibiotics. Penicillin or amoxicillin given for ten days is the treatment of choice.

Strep throat is uncommon under three years of age and is usually not accompanied by a cough or runny nose. There is often a fever, a very sore throat, headache, abdominal pain and sometimes vomiting. The throat and tonsils are red, there may be little red spots over the palate (roof of the mouth) and there is often yellow pus on the tonsils.

The lymph glands on each side of the neck become swollen and tender. Some streptococcal germs produce a toxin which causes a red skin rash. This rash spares the face, and is mainly over the trunk in the warm areas such as groin and armpits. It feels bumpy like sand paper. If the rash is present the disease is called scarlet fever or scarlatina (if the fever is low-grade only).

A "rapid strep test" can be used by the doctor in the office to see if the streptococcus is present in the throat.

It is important to treat strep throat for a full 10 days with antibiotics to prevent a complication called rheumatic fever (which luckily is quite rare today) that sometimes occurs in untreated strep throat.

Some children (and adults) do not respond to medication. These people are "strep carriers." They have a few of the streptococcus germs living in their throat, but are not sick from them. If a strep carrier later gets a viral sore throat and is tested with a rapid strep test or a throat culture, the test will be positive even though a virus is causing the illness. Treatment will not improve these patients.

Best Advice:

If your child has a sore throat with cold and cough, it is probably caused by a virus and antibiotics will not help. Sore throats with fever, swollen glands, a skin rash or marked tiredness should be checked by your doctor. Always have your child take all the medication your doctor prescribes, even if he or she is better in a few days. Removal of the tonsils (tonsillectomy) is almost never necessary.

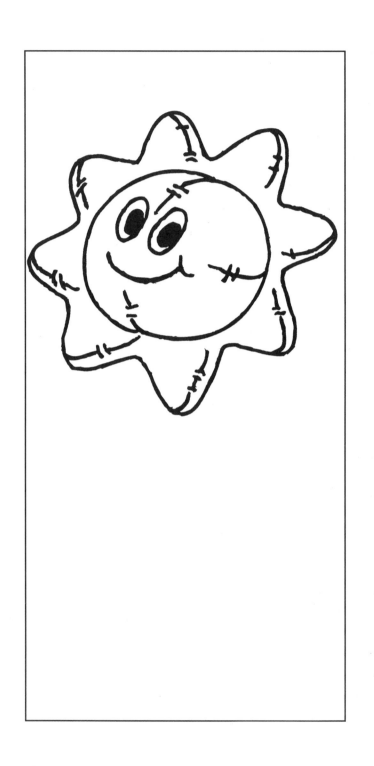

Thirteen

Teaching the Birds and the Bees

Talking about sex is difficult for most parents. Always tell the truth. If you are not truthful, your child will not trust you later on.

Start early

With little children, do not go into any great detail. They want only a brief one- or two-sentence answer to satisfy their immediate question.

Use the opportunities in your surroundings. Sex education is a slow, ongoing process from toddler to teenager. When your toddler asks about a fat, pregnant neighbor or relative, give a simple answer. "She has a baby in her tummy" usually satisfies and teaches. To the question, "How does it get there," answer "It grows there." "How does the baby get out?" "The mother pushes it out." This simple exchange is a good start at sex education.

Use proper names in describing parts and functions of the body.

Rather than an official talk, use opportunities as they arise and slowly, over the years, explain the basics. For example, if a local pet has babies, visit with your child and use this opportunity to continue your training. In this way your child will learn that you are willing to discuss the subject openly and to answer questions honestly. The child will both learn and realize that talking about sex is not forbidden or secret.

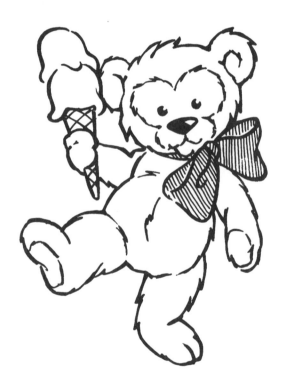

Fourteen

The Early School Years

Bicycle helmets

Bicycle helmets reduce the risk of serious head injury by 85 percent. Helmets should be worn each time your child rides a bike. Get one; it is money well spent and in many places the law requires the wearing of a helmet.

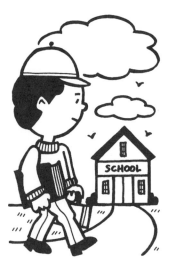

Skateboards and in-line skates

These are great fun, but dangerous. Injuries to the arms, legs, head and neck are common. Do not let a child below five years of age skateboard or use in-line skates. Their motor coordination and judgment are not good enough.

Insist that your child use a protective helmet and elbow and knee pads. Never let your child skate in the street or on the highway. Only the sidewalk or driveway are safe.

School readiness

When your child is approaching school age, the question may come up: Should I send my child to school or wait another year? Also after kindergarten: Is my child ready for first grade? Many children are considered immature by their nursery or preschool teachers. They are tested, and the recommendation is made to parents: Hold the child back for social-interaction reasons.

Here is what is known (you may not hear this from your friends or the school system):

- Children who are younger in first grade have a slightly lower achievement rate, but that disappears by third grade.

- The youngest kindergarten child always has a slight disadvantage.

- The child that you voluntarily hold back is often not challenged enough so he or she may actually do worse.

- The tests that check for school readiness were designed to help teachers plan instruction. *None is accurate enough to screen for school readiness.* There is as much as a 50 percent error rate.

Kindergarten and first-grade retention:
- By the time children have completed first grade, "repeaters" do *not* outperform comparison students.

- They do feel more negative about school.

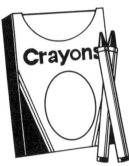

There is often no achievement benefit in retaining children in kindergarten or first grade. Regardless of how well you explain the extra year to the child, it may still have an emotional cost.

Best Advice:

Your child goes to school to learn, only secondarily to socialize. A little immaturity is common and will no longer be noticeable by third grade. It is probably not wise to hold a normal child back.

Team sports

Team sports, such as soccer and football are good for children. They teach sportsmanship and how to get along with others.

You as a parent must do your homework before you sign up your child. Meet and spend some time talking to the coach:

- Does the coach stress winning, or that the children have fun and learn?

- Will your child get to participate rather than always sitting on the bench?

- Does the coach encourage children to play if injured, "for the good of the team"?

- Will there be a proper warm-up period?

Check all of this before you allow your child to join the team.

Best Advice:

Sports should be fun for children, and a good program tries to achieve this. Most important: Do not get mad at your child if his or her performance is less than you expected.

Eye exercises

Eye exercises are periodically in the news. Some optometrists prescribe these to help your child move his or her eyes smoothly together and to improve vision, athletics and reading skills.

Your child's school may suggest that your child needs eye exercises to improve coordination, balance, reading, or learning.

Parents with clumsy children and children who are not reading well want to help their children do better. They become convinced that eye exercises are useful and needlessly spend large amounts of money in multiple visits to their practitioner's office.

There is no evidence that eye exercises do what is claimed or that they are of any value. The exercises may help some children because the child gets extra attention. You can do this better and more cheaply by spending time with your child, rather than paying someone else a lot of money to do it.

Best Advice:

Always check with your doctor or qualified ophthalmologist if teachers or friends recommend that your child needs these exercises to improve reading or coordination.

Reading

Teach your child that reading is wonderful. There are thousands of marvelous stories available in books. Reading to younger children is time well-spent for both parent and child.

Encourage some reading daily, before you turn on the TV. The love of reading is a gift that your child will treasure forever.

Best Advice:

Children imitate parents, so keep books, magazines and newspapers around your house, and you read, too.

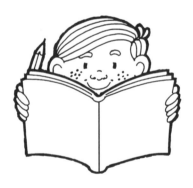

Fifteen

Puberty

The physical changes in normal children at puberty occur in an orderly fashion and over a definite time frame. The age when puberty starts varies with general health, nutrition, genetics and the family's socioeconomic status.

Girls

Breast development is under hormonal control. While full breast development usually does not start until the girl is about eleven years old, around eight years of age some little girls find small, tender buttons of breast tissue right under one or both nipples. These small lumps are little breast-buds, sensitive to the small amounts of female sex hormones put out at this age. These breast-buds do not get very large and may stay or go away.

Girls experiencing this need lots of reassurance that this is normal. It must be stressed that they do not have cancer and that their breasts will not get much bigger for a fairly long time. Because extra blood flows through these breast buttons, the breasts are extra tender and may hurt if the girl bumps into something. This is nothing to worry about.

It is very important that these breast-buds are recognized for what they are. The buds must not be removed surgically by a doctor mistaking them for something serious such as cancer. If removed, there will be no normal breast development in that location ever.

True puberty in girls usually starts between nine and fifteen years of age. There is a growth-spurt of several years and fat is laid down, changing the girl's shape. Real breast development begins and axillary and pubic hair starts to grow. This hair is caused by androgen (male sex hormone), a little of which is present in all girls.

Two to three years into this growth spurt menstrual periods begin. This usually happens between eleven and eighteen years of age and is a normal part of growing up.

It is important that you explain to your pre-teen daughter that menstruation is going to happen, and what to do when it does. The teenager must understand that it is a normal process and not dangerous. She must be prepared in case her periods start when she is away from home. You must teach her about sanitary napkins (pads) and tampons.

Menstruation is often very irregular for the first two to three years after periods start. In most young women menstruation (periods) then comes fairly regularly, on a monthly basis, but may be only every two to three months in some. It is recommended that women have at least four or more periods a year. If your teenage daughter has fewer periods check with your doctor.

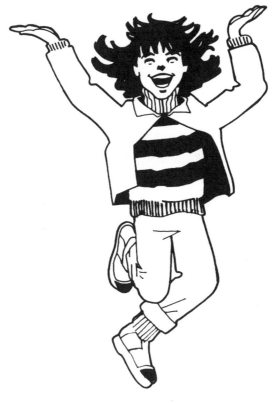

Protection: external or internal? It is a good idea to start your daughter out on sanitary napkins. But there is nothing wrong with teaching her how to use tampons, which will make her life much easier. Tampons are OK at any age, as long as the girl can get them in. It is important that tampons not be worn for twenty-four hours because of the risk of toxic shock (a serious condition caused by bacteria growing in the tampon). As long as tampons are changed every five to eight hours and are not worn during the night, there should be no problem.

Menstrual cramps are common, especially in the first few years after periods start. Cramps are easier to prevent than to treat. Exercise works well at making cramps better. If medication is needed, over-the-counter drugs such as Advil or Motrin (ibuprofen) and Aleve (naproxen) are very effective. Taken early, this group of drugs works better than many over-the-counter cramp medications.

For the first few years after periods start, young girls may not ovulate every month, and sometimes have many days of heavy bleeding. This can usually be treated with iron pills from the drugstore. If the bleeding is very heavy and continues, your doctor may want to start your daughter on birth control pills for three to four months. This use of "the pill" is as a medicine and not for birth control and usually works well.

Menstrual periods are no reason not to go to school, take part in athletic events, or in any way change your daughter's lifestyle.

Boys

Puberty in boys usually starts two years later than in girls. First the penis, scrotum (sack) and testicles start to grow, followed shortly by pubic hair. Then rapid growth starts. During this time, the circulating hormones stimulate the larynx (voice box), causing it to grow. This causes the Adam's apple to protrude. The vocal cords

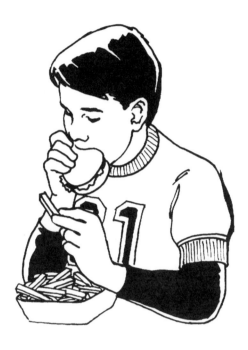

lengthen and the voice will break, changing from high to low, sometimes in mid-sentence. Eventually the voice will permanently deepen.

Axillary and facial hair usually appear two years after pubic hair starts to grow. Night time ejaculation starts about one year after the penis starts growing. This is normal.

Many boys have some breast development around puberty. This is called gynecomastia. It occurs in 30 to 50 percent of all boys. It is caused by estrogen (the female sex hormone), present in small amounts in all males. These breast lumps are tender, do not get very large, and usually go away after several years. Teenage boys need a lot of reassurance that this is normal.

The boy must understand that this is not cancer, that the breasts will not get large enough to cause a problem, and that many of his friends also have gynecomastia.

Occasionally a boy who develops large breasts will be so worried about his looks that it causes psychological difficulty. These boys refuse to go swimming, will not undress if others are present, and withdraw emotionally. Professional counseling and/or evaluation by a plastic surgeon for cosmetic removal may be necessary.

Best Advice:

Puberty is a stressful time for parents and children. Hormones are raging just as new vistas open up.

It takes a lot of love, cooperation and tolerance on both sides for the family structure to survive in the best condition.

Sixteen

Teenagers!

Teenagers take a lot of work but can also be a lot of fun.

Behavioral patterns are imprinted in the first five to seven years of life. It was during these growing years when your child's morals, ethics and overall philosophy of life were implanted. Now is the time to reinforce these teachings.

The teenage years are a turbulent time. There are hormonal swings, peer pressure, and the teenager's need to establish an identity separate from that of his or her parents.

The home and family will be less important as the teenager ventures out into the world. Conformity with the group and friends now play a larger part in the teenager's life.

Teenagers eat lots of junk food but they are still growing, so provide a good multivitamin with minerals to make sure they get the nutrients they need.

The teenager is at times a child, at others an adult. It is important to remember teenagers, despite their rebelliousness, desperately need boundaries and rules to govern their behavior. They will fight these rules, but are lost without them.

They are old enough to discuss decisions that concern them and the family, but they really want the parent to be in charge. Teenagers are not comfortable or secure if they can do whatever they want.

Discipline

It helps to sit down with the teenager when everything is calm, before there is conflict. Discuss what you as parents expect and what punishments or rewards may come into play.

Together with your child, make a set of basic rules. These should cover:

- Behavior at home and in public

- School and after-school sports and activities

- The possibility of employment after school, on weekends and during vacations

- Involvement with friends and peers

- Use of the telephone and car

Listen to the teenager's complaints, desires and concerns and see if you can incorporate some of his or her ideas and suggestions. Determine together what will happen if these rules are broken.

Write it all down and make three copies that everybody signs. One copy is for you, one for the teenager, and one to be kept on the refrigerator. This way the rules are in place before conflict arises.

Best Advice:

Do not make new rules while having an argument with your teenager.

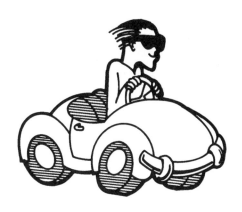

Driving

It is great to have a teenager always ready and willing to drive the car to run your errands. Just make sure your teenager knows the rules of the road and what you as parents expect from a teenage driver.

Judiciously use the car as "carrot and stick" to modify behavior.

Make the teenager responsible for helping to pay for gas and, if there is an income from work, for some of the insurance.

Drugs, alcohol, tobacco

Talk to your teenager about the dangers of drugs, alcohol, and smoking or other tobacco use. Always set a good example. Remember, you are a role model for your teenager.

Drinking and driving do not mix. Make a pact with your teenager: In a situation where the driver has been drinking (your teenager or someone else), it takes only one telephone call for you, the parent, to come, no questions asked, to bring the teenager home. You can discuss the situation later, when everyone has cooled down.

Sex

Teen pregnancy and sexually transmitted diseases are, unfortunately, a fact of life today. Acquired Immune Deficiency Syndrome (AIDS) is spreading in this age group.

Talk to your teenager about sex, birth control and how to prevent sexually transmitted disease. The life you save may be your child's.

Acne

The cause of acne is unknown. There are many sebaceous glands on the face, back and chest. With acne these glands become plugged. This causes white heads, black heads and redness (inflammation).

- Eighty-five percent of all people (boys and girls) have some acne.

- Acne is not dangerous and almost always goes away eventually.

- For the teenager for whom looks are very important, acne is a catastrophe.

- Acne seems to run in families.

- Acne appears between nine and seventeen years of age when sexual maturity occurs.

If inflammation is severe, cysts may form. Acne gets worse during times of stress and with menstrual periods.

Diet is probably not a cause, but if some foods seem to make it worse, these foods should be avoided.

Acne is a long-term problem and there are no quick cures. Cleanliness helps. Treat the face gently when you wash. Do not pick the pimples. That may cause permanent scars.

There are several ways to treat acne, but it may take weeks or months before you see improvement. Be patient and give the treatment a chance.

Topical Medications:
- Benzoyl peroxide. This effective medication is available at the drugstore without a prescription as Oxy-5, Oxy-10 or Clearasil. It works quite well. Prescription strength benzoyl peroxide comes as a cream or gel, and is more effective.

- Retin-A. This medication is available by prescription only. It works very well but may be irritating. It is applied once a day or every other day, depending on how red the skin gets from its use.

- Topical antibiotics. Also available by prescription only are liquid clindamycin and liquid erythromycin. Both work well to control the redness.

Topical treatment often combines two or more of these medications. If after nine to sixteen weeks of topical treatment the acne is no better, medication by mouth is necessary.

Oral Medications:
- Tetracycline or erythromycin. These prescription drugs are antibiotics given in small daily doses and work very well for many teenagers. The redness disappears and the acne improves. After years of experience we know that long term use of these medications causes no side effects. Remember that tetracycline must be taken on an empty stomach and not with milk.

- Accutane. If the acne persists and is very severe, this prescription drug may be used. It is taken by mouth for three months and occasionally causes severe side effects. Accutane does cure most cases of acne. It is available only from a dermatologist.

Best Advice:

With a little luck and a lot of work, your teenager will be a person you can both love and respect.

Remember that despite the turbulence often experienced during these years most parents and children do survive.

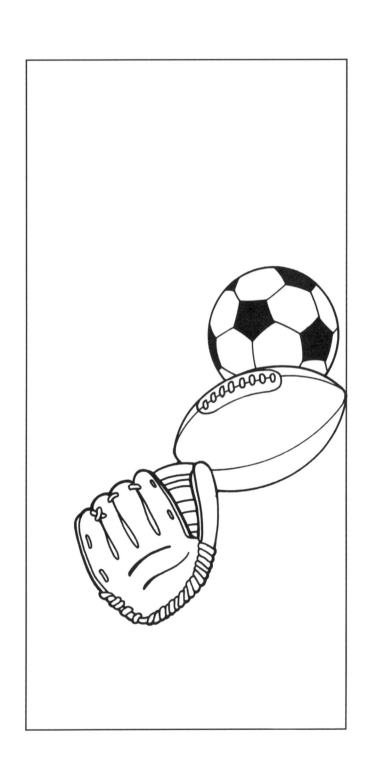

Seventeen

Common Health Concerns — All Ages

Abdominal pain (stomachache)

Bellyaches are very common in children. They often continue, on and off, for months or years. Some bellyaches are caused by serious illnesses such as appendicitis or a bladder or kidney infection. This serious type of bellyache usually gets rapidly worse and there may be other symptoms such as weight loss, vomiting, diarrhea, frequent painful urination, and loss of appetite. The child looks ill (see How to Tell if Your Child is Really Ill, page 21). Consult your doctor immediately.

The closer the child points to the bellybutton, when you ask where the pain is, the less likely it is that the bellyache is caused by something serious.

The bellyache that is long-lasting, mildly painful, nagging, and comes and goes is a different problem. This condition has been called chronic abdominal pain, mucus colitis, spastic colitis, and functional bowel distress. It really worries parents. We do not know what causes these bellyaches. However, the children usually eat well, are quite happy, go to school, and generally look healthy.

Chronic abdominal pain is a diagnosis by exclusion. In other words, the doctor has to make sure that there is nothing serious going on. If your child has a long-lasting bellyache, a visit to the doctor is necessary. A blood count, urine, and possibly some stool samples need to be checked. The chances of finding something serious are slim, but your doctor has to make sure that nothing serious is causing the pain.

Here are some simple things you can try:

- See if there is any stress in the child's life that you can ease. Is something going on at home or in school that bothers the child? Is there too much involvement in outside activities such as sports or music lessons? Try to make the child's life a little easier.

- Sometimes an over-the-counter medication such as Maalox Plus helps.

- A medication called Donnatal (this has to be prescribed by your doctor) may help.

Many of these bellyaches last for years, reoccurring intermittently in spite of everything that may be done. As the child gets older, though the pain may persist, it becomes less important in the child's life.

Best Advice:

Chronic abdominal pain is common in children. If your doctor says there is nothing serious going on, some simple measures may help to make the child more comfortable.

Appendicitis

Like gastroenteritis (see Vomiting and diarrhea, page 170), appendicitis starts with a bellyache. The pain is mild and throughout the belly, then gradually gets worse. After several hours, it moves and settles in the right side. Nausea and vomiting are common, but usually there is no diarrhea.

Children with appendicitis may have a normal temperature or run a little fever (99°-101° F). They are not hungry and do not want to eat. With viral gastroenteritis, the child varies between feeling better and worse, but the child with appendicitis gets progressively worse.

Appendicitis is a clinical diagnosis, and blood counts or X-rays help only a little.

Appendicitis is common after five years of age, and any child with a bellyache and vomiting should be closely watched.

Appendicitis does occur in the two- to three-year-old, but is difficult to diagnose before rupture. Check with your doctor if your child is vomiting and has a loss of appetite.

Best Advice:

Appendicitis is very serious and occurs during the flu season as well as at other times of the year. Consider it a possibility regardless of what virus is making its way through the community.

Any bellyache which gets worse, especially if there is vomiting and loss of appetite, is appendicitis until proven otherwise. Call your doctor.

Asthma

Many children wheeze in the first few years of life. Asthma is the most common chronic childhood disease.

Asthma is a condition in which the bronchioles (small tubes in the lungs), through which we breathe, become temporarily narrowed or blocked due to various "triggers."

This is what happens: When the trigger irritates the bronchioles, they tighten up and narrow. Mucus enters and causes more narrowing. This is what causes breathing difficulties. The child inhales and has difficulty breathing the air back out. This makes the wheezing sound.

Everyone's airway reacts to irritants, but the airway in asthmatics is supersensitive (more easily and more severely irritated).

Heredity is a risk factor: Asthmatic parents often have asthmatic children.

Common triggers:

- Allergies do not cause asthma, but they can trigger an attack.

- Viral or bacterial infections are common triggers.

- Tobacco smoke, paint fumes and perfume are well-known triggers.

- Exercise often acts as a trigger.

- Cold air acts as a trigger. This is why asthma attacks often start and get worse at night.

Treating asthma is complicated. Removing the trigger is important and then the broncho-spasm and inflammation must be relieved. The bronchodilators albuterol or adrenalin are pre-scription medications which help to relax the muscles in spasm around the bronchioles.

Bronchodilators can be given by mouth, as pills or liquid, or by injection. They are then car-ried to the lungs by way of the blood stream. They also can be inhaled directly into the lungs. Inhalation is the preferred route. A smaller amount is needed since the medication is deliv-ered directly to the lungs and this results in fewer side effects, the most common of which are rapid heart beat and jitteriness.

Cromolyn and steroids (cortisone) are pre-ventative medications for asthma. Both are anti-inflammatory medications that help to decrease the mucus and swelling inside the bronchioles. Cromolyn and steroids have to be inhaled several times a day and do not work to relieve an acute asthmatic attack. They are available by prescription only.

Often a combination of medications is necessary to successfully treat asthma.

Goals of treatment are:

- To provide restful sleep at night.

- To avoid hospitalization and emergency room visits

- To allow the child to play with friends and go to school regularly.

- To help the child lead a normal, happy, active life.

(See also Croup, page 85; and Epiglottitis page 88)

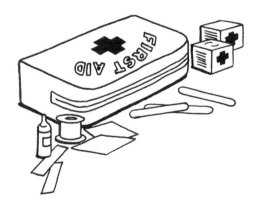

Bites, animal

If an animal bites your child and the wound is small:
- Wash the wound with lots of water.

- Check your child's immunization status: Is tetanus up to date?

- Try to identify the biting animal and check if it has had its rabies vaccine.

- Call and talk with your doctor.

If the wound is large and appears serious, call your doctor immediately or take your child to an emergency room. The animal must be confined and watched for fourteen days to make sure it does not have rabies. Confinement is necessary even in vaccinated animals. If the animal is not available for observation, discuss other options with your doctor.

Bites from domestic rodents (rabbits, guinea pigs, hamsters, rats) must be watched for infection, but these animals usually do not carry rabies.

Bats, skunks, and raccoons are known rabies carriers. These animals are dangerous. Keep your child away from them and from any animal, wild or pet, which appears ill.

Animal bites are dirty and easily get infected. Antibiotics are usually needed, so check with your doctor.

(See also Bites, human, below)

Best Advice:

A pet animal gets only one bite. Do not keep an animal in your house once it has bitten a child. Regardless of how long you have had the pet, get rid of it.

Bites, human

Human bites are fairly common and are more dangerous than most animal bites. The human mouth is dirtier and has more (and worse) bacteria than most animal mouths. Any human bite that breaks the skin should probably be reported to your doctor, who may want to start antibiotics to prevent infection.

Best Advice:

Always worry about a human bite, even a little one. Check with your doctor and watch the bite area closely until healed.

Bites and stings, insects

Insect stings hurt first and then become red, swollen, and itchy. As soon as possible, cover the sting area with a paste of meat-tenderizer and water, or baking soda and water, or soap and water. If none of these is readily available, cover the area with spit. With bee stings, make sure that you remove the stinger first; otherwise more of the poison will be forced into the stung area.

Bee and wasp stings often continue to swell, redden, and itch for two to three days. This does not mean that they are infected, and they do get better after a few days.

Benadryl (diphenhydramine hydrochloride) from the drugstore, taken by mouth, often relieves the swelling and itching.

To minimize the chances of insect bites, make sure your child wears shoes and long-sleeved shirts when he or she is playing outside. You can buy good spray-on insect repellents at the drugstore. Vitamin B-1 (thiamin), 100-200 milligrams taken daily during the summer months, gives a faint smell to the skin that most insects detest. This smell keeps mosquitoes and many other insects away.

Bleeding

Cuts and abrasions are common injuries in children and often are accompanied by some bleeding.

You cannot evaluate the damage if everything is covered with blood, so the first thing to do is to stop the bleeding. Some areas of the body bleed more than others because more blood vessels are near the surface and so more get broken. These areas are the face, scalp and genitalia.

When the skin and underlying blood vessels are broken, the blood vessels contract, and platelets (small particles in the blood) stick to the edges and form a plug, closing the vessel opening. Then fibrin in the blood is activated to form a stable, more permanent clot.

When there is bleeding, elevate the bleeding area. Apply firm pressure with a *dry* cloth for several minutes. A wet cloth will not stop bleeding. Almost all bleeding will stop and you can see the injury better. Many cuts and abrasions don't look so bad when bleeding has stopped, and a simple antibiotic ointment (Neosporin or Polysporin) may be all that is necessary.

Cuts inside the mouth and on the tongue bleed a lot. It is hard to apply pressure, so for this type of bleeding encourage your child to suck on ice chips. The cold helps to contract the blood vessels so a clot forms and the bleeding stops.

Best Advice:

Stop bleeding with firm pressure. Then evaluate the injury and call your doctor if it looks serious.

Bronchitis
(cough)

If your child has a persistent cough and does not have a pneumonia, it is called bronchitis (inflammation of the bronchial tubes in the lungs). There are many causes for bronchitis.

Viral bronchitis is common. Antibiotics do not help and the disease (cough) has to run its course.

Mycoplasma bronchitis occurs in older children and teenagers. This bronchitis gets better faster if an antibiotic, usually erythromycin, is used. The child is moderately sick but up and about. There may be a low-grade fever. This type of bronchitis is closely related to what is called walking pneumonia.

Allergic bronchitis is also common. This bronchitis is caused by an inhalant allergy (pollen in the air that the child breathes) and may last a long time, until the pollen causing the allergy is gone. It is quite similar to asthma (the asthmatic cough is an allergic cough). The same medications used for asthma are used and often help.

Asthmatic bronchitis is also an allergic bronchitis, but with some wheezing associated with the cough.

Quite often the child also will have a bacterial or viral infection in the ears, throat, sinuses or lungs. This infection gets the bronchitis started. Antibiotics may be needed to cure this infection; otherwise the bronchitis will not go away.

Allergic—or rarely, infectious—sinusitis (inflammation of the sinuses) can cause a postnasal drip that runs down into the lungs (especially when the child lies down). The child coughs to get this mucus back out of the lungs. This cough is usually worse at night.

Most bronchitis coughs sound the same, and may be quite difficult to sort out. Children do not cough and spit, but cough and swallow, so you will see little of the material that is coughed up.

Treatment includes:

- Humidification. Humidify the air with a cold-mist humidifier. (A hot steam vaporizer works as well but is dangerous since if the child pulls the unit over, the hot water may cause severe burns.) Or, if nothing else is available, run the shower on hot and let the child inhale the steam for a few minutes.

- Expectorant cough medicine. This loosens mucus and makes coughing more effective.

- Specific medicine. Antibiotics or antiallergy medication, depending on the cause, may help.

Best Advice:

If your child has a cough, feels well, and has no fever, you can safely treat it at home. If there is a fever or if the cough lasts many weeks, a visit to the doctor is necessary.

Burns

Small, superficial skin burns are common and heal without scarring. Immediately soak the burned area in cool water. Do not use ice (it can cause further skin damage). If blisters form, do not pop them. The skin will heal better with the blister intact. Any large burn or burn on the palm, sole or the genitals is potentially serious and needs urgent medical attention.

Canker sores

Canker sores afflict both children and adults. They are small, yellow ulcers in the mouth, gums, and throat. They are very painful, but your child will not be ill.

Canker sores are caused by a virus that, once the child is infected, lives indefinitely in the cells of his or her mouth. As mouth resistance goes down, out come the canker sores. When mouth resistance goes up, the sores disappear. There is little that helps.

What you can do:
- Do not give acid food and fluid (like orange juice). Give your child

cold, bland, good-tasting foods and fluids instead.

- Use Tylenol (acetaminophen) for pain relief.

- Your doctor can prescribe liquid xylocaine. This is a local anesthetic and gives relief, but tastes so awful that most children (and adults) would rather hurt that use it.

- You can buy liquid Benadryl (diphenhydramine hydrochloride) at the drugstore. Rinsing the mouth with it helps a little.

- You can buy liquid Maalox at the drugstore. Rinsing the mouth with it helps a little. (A combination of Benadryl and Maalox works fairly well).

Remember, canker sores eventually always go away by themselves.

There are several diseases with canker-sore-like mouth ulcers. A sore throat with fever, possibly vomiting, and bellyache occurs with a coxsacki virus infection. The ulcers are over only the back of the throat and the child is generally ill. This disease lasts for seven to ten days and clears by itself. Treat with Tylenol (acetaminophen) and cold, good-tasting fluids and food.

Hand, foot, mouth disease causes ulcers

over the throat and the palms and soles of the feet. (See Hand, foot, mouth disease, page 147)

Herpetiform gingivostomatitis is an infection with the herpes 1 virus. There is a high fever and the child's gums become red, swollen, and start to bleed. The teeth may become loose. Whitish ulcers appear all over the mouth, including the tongue, gums and throat. Children with this infection are truly miserable. The disease can last from a few days to several weeks and there is little you can do except use Tylenol (acetaminophen) and use your wits to get enough food and fluids into the child to keep body and soul together.

The good news: Herpetiform gingivostomatitis always heals itself. The gums will return to normal, the bleeding will stop, and the teeth will become firm again. No permanent damage occurs. It is a miserable disease, but everything will turn out all right.

Colds

Colds (runny nose, with an occasional cough and minimal fever, also called upper respiratory tract infections or URIs) are caused by a number of viruses. Colds do not need (and do not get better with) antibiotics, so do not ask your doctor for one.

You can make a good nose drop:

1 cup of water

1/4 teaspoon salt.

Put four or five drops in each nostril every three to four hours.

A cold-mist humidifier at night helps colds and coughs. Hot steam vaporizers do the same, but if they spill, they often cause burns.

Cold weather injuries

Cold weather injuries such as frostbite occur if the face, nose, ears, hands and feet are not kept warm and dry. There is little padding in these areas to protect the skin and underlying cells from cold exposure. The small blood vessels clot and later ice crystals form in the tissues. The skin becomes red and then pale as the blood stops flowing. On rewarming, the skin becomes red and blisters may form.

Treatment consists of rapid warming of the affected body parts. Do not massage the skin or rub snow or ice into the area. Prevent infection if blisters form. Recovery is usually quite good.

Best Advice:
Prevent cold weather injuries by dressing your child properly. Make sure that hands, nose, ears and feet stay warm and dry when your child is out playing in the cold.

Cuts and bruises

Cuts and bruises are usually minor and

need little care. Wash them with soap and water and keep them clean and dry. An over-the-counter antibiotic ointment (Neosporin or Polysporin), applied several times a day, helps prevent cuts from becoming infected. Cuts over one-half inch long or gaping wounds may need stitches. Have your doctor check them.

Eyelid infections (sties)

Sties are common in children and teenagers. This is what happens: One of the small glands along the rim of the eyelid opens up and becomes infected with bacteria that happen to be on the eyelid.

Once the gland is infected, there is redness, swelling and tenderness. A little boil forms at the edge of the eyelid by the eyelashes. This is called a "sty." The boil has to pop and drain before the infection can heal. The pus that comes out of the boil contains more bacteria and is smeared along both eyelids by the child's hands. When the next gland opens, the process repeats itself and another sty forms. This can go on for months. Always carefully wash the child's and your hands after touching the eyes.

Treatment consists of hot soaks and an antibiotic ointment your doctor will prescribe rubbed into the eyelashes several times a day. Sometimes, if caught early, oral antibiotics may prevent boil formation.

Best Advice:

At the first sign of eyelid swelling or redness, start hot compresses (a warm, wet cloth placed on the affected area) and see your doctor for a prescription for an antibiotic eye ointment. Continue rubbing the ointment sparingly into the eyelashes once or twice daily for several weeks after the sty is gone to kill all the bacteria and prevent recurrence.

Fever

With fevers, it is important to remember:

- It's not the fever you worry about, but what causes the fever.

- Your child can be very sick with a low fever, and not very sick with a high fever.

- Any baby under three months of age with a temperature of 100.8° F or more must be seen by a doctor!

- High fever by itself (even up to 106° F) does not cause brain damage.

- High fever may cause a fever convulsion in babies six months to three years of age.

- The best way to lower fever is to use Tylenol (acetaminophen), or Advil or Motrin (ibuprofen).

- Aspirin, though it works well, is not recommended and should not be used because of the possibility that it may cause Reyes Syndrome, a very serious complication, in some children.

Give your fever-lowering medication every three and a half to four hours to keep the fever down.

These medications take thirty to forty minutes to start bringing fever down. The fever may continue to rise during this period. Luke warm baths help a little, and keep you busy while you wait for the fever-lowering medications to work. *Never* use ice-water or alcohol baths.

Most fevers are caused by viruses which have to run their course.

(See also Fever convulsions page 89)

Best Advice:

If your baby looks ill, regardless of his or her temperature, call your doctor.

Fifth disease (slapped cheek disease)

This is an infection caused by a Parvo virus. There may be fever and a fine, delicate rash over face, body, arms, and legs. The cheeks are often a bright, shiny red and the reason for the name "slapped cheek disease." This illness lasts for five to ten days, but the rash may come and go for several weeks. Treatment consists of fever control.

Though harmless to your child, this virus occasionally causes birth defects, and you should keep your little one away from women who may be newly pregnant.

Fungus infections of the skin (ringworm, athlete's foot, jockstrap itch)

Fungus infections are common in children. There are many fungi in the environment, and they cause different skin diseases. A fungus is not a bacterium and so does not respond to antibiotics. There are several antifungal medications available, and some of these can be bought without a prescription.

Fungi invade the top layer of skin and live there. They especially like moist, dark places and grow in the diaper area, genital area of girls and athletes, and on the skin of sweaty feet.

Monilial diaper rash (see Diaper rash, page 41) is a fungus infection.

Ringworm can be on the scalp or on the body. Scalp ringworm starts with a small, red area which slowly grows.

Soon there is scaling, crusting and the hairs break off, causing a partially bald area. This has to be distinguished from alopecia areata, a condition of unknown cause which results in bald spots on the scalp. With alopecia areata, the hair is completely gone and not broken off at various lengths, as with ringworm. Ringworm also must be distinguished from hair-pulling by nervous children who literally pull their hair out in spots, often as they are going to sleep.

Sometimes scalp ringworm becomes infected with bacteria. Then a raised, pussy red area forms. This is called a kerion and must be treated with antibiotics and antifungal medication. Scalp ringworm needs to be checked by a doctor as a prescription for oral medication (griseofulvin) is necessary along with local treatment. Local treatment can be with an antifungal cream or Selsun Blue brand shampoo.

Ringworm on the body starts as a red spot that is dry and scaly and spreads in a circle (red rim and pale, scaly inside). Your child can get this ringworm from a cat, dog or another child and it will spread over the body if not treated. Body ringworm has to be distinguished from nummular (coin-shaped) eczema and impetigo. Treatment consists of an antifungal ointment. Clotrimazole (Mycelex, Lotrimin) and miconazole (Micatin) work well.

Ringworm in the genital area is called "jockstrap itch." A red spot forms which spreads, causing a reddish-brown area with a red, slightly raised border. This form of ringworm is common in athletes and others who sweat a lot and wear tight underwear. Treatment consists of wearing loose garments, blow-drying the area with warm air after baths or exercise, and one of the anti-fungal ointments.

Fungus infections of the feet, called athlete's foot, spreads from person to person. There is redness and scaling of the skin. Cracks and crusts form between the toes, and there is an intense itch. You can treat this infection yourself. Change the child's socks frequently, keep the feet dry (you can dry them with a blow-dryer set on "warm") and use an antifungal medication. For athlete's foot Tinactin (tolnaftate) or Desenex work well.

Reinfection is common. If your child's feet do not improve with this treatment, the child probably does not have athlete's foot but has a foot allergy. An allergic reaction can occur in children who wear tennis or other shoes with a glued-on sole. Sweat from the feet dissolves some of the glue, which can trigger the allergy. There is generalized scaling and itching, but the cracks and crusts between the toes are missing. Treatment consists of having the child stop wearing sneakers. Most children and teenagers will tolerate some discomfort to continue to wear sneakers like their peers. An over-the-counter cortisone cream (Cortaid or Cortizone-10) helps a little. As the child ages there will be less sweating and the condition will clear up.

Best Advice:

Fungus infections are common and are not caused by dirt. Fungi grow best in dark, damp places so conditions caused by fungi get better with fresh air, dryness and the application of one of the nonprescription antifungal medications.

Any skin condition that does not improve over two to three weeks should be checked by a doctor.

Hand, foot and mouth disease

This is a viral infection, which usually occurs in the spring and fall. Symptoms consist of fever and little blisters on a red background. These blisters occur on the hands and soles of the feet, and there are little ulcers (like canker sores) in the mouth and throat. The child does not feel well, does not want to eat and is cranky.

There is no treatment. Fluids, fever control with Tylenol (acetaminophen) and time will make the child better.

Head injuries

Children continually fall or bump into objects and hurt their heads. Head injuries are usually minor and not serious.

Almost immediately a swelling forms on the forehead or scalp where the injury occurred.

This bluish pooching-out is caused by blood collecting between the skin and the bone. If there is no confusion, loss of memory, or loss of consciousness, this is nothing to worry about. It is a bruise and will go away over a few days.

If the head injury is more severe, the brain may be hurt. This is called a concussion. There may be headache, vomiting, confusion, loss of memory and loss of consciousness.

You must watch any child with a head injury carefully for at least twenty-four hours to make sure that there are no changes in mental status.

Concussions range from mild to serious:

- Mild concussion: There is no loss of consciousness, no loss of memory, but the child may be briefly confused. This child must be watched closely for twenty-four hours for *any* changes in behavior. An hour after the injury the child can return to normal activity.

- Moderate concussion: There is no loss of consciousness, but some loss of memory and the child is confused. Call your doctor to ask whether the child should be seen. There may be vomiting. Keep the child quiet and watch closely for twenty-four hours (wake the child hourly during the night). Look for any change in alertness and behavior. Keep the child out of strenuous activity for one week.

- Severe concussion: There is loss of consciousness. This is an emergency. Call an ambulance or take the child to an emergency room.

Best Advice:

Most head injuries are not serious but the child must be watched for twenty-four hours. If there is vomiting, confusion, memory loss or loss of consciousness, call your doctor!

Headaches

Headaches probably occur early in life, but we cannot tell until the child lets us know. In the toddler, generalized bacterial or viral infections are a common cause of headache.

After five years of age, headaches become more common.

Some things to note:

- Eyes almost never cause headaches.

- Sinuses almost never cause headaches in infants or toddlers.

We can break children's headaches into

three main categories, organic, vascular, and tension.

Organic headaches

There is something extra in the head taking up space. A brain tumor, cyst, blood-vessel abnormality or water on the brain (hydrocephalus) can cause this pain.

This headache is due to pressure. It is present in the morning, may last all day and often the child vomits without being nauseated. Vomiting may make the child feel better for a little while. Headaches caused by pressure get progressively worse until the cause is removed.

These headaches are very rare. Any persistent morning headache, especially if there is vomiting, needs urgent medical attention.

Vascular headaches

These bad headaches include migraine headaches. The pain is severe, throbbing, episodic and often associated with nausea and vomiting. The pain may be on one or both sides of the head. Pain medications work somewhat, but resting in a dark room and sleeping for a few hours gives the most relief. Once the pain goes away, the child is completely well, until the next headache starts.

Vascular headaches run in families. The pain is caused by blood vessels in the brain which open and narrow. In most patients, over-the-counter pain medication such as Tylenol (acetaminophen) and rest is the treatment of choice. If there are many attacks, daily preventive medications prescribed by your doctor often work.

Tension headaches

These headaches are very common in children. The headache feels like pressure or a band around the head.

Tension headaches come and go, but never completely go away. The child will tell you the headache is always sort of there in the background. This headache gets worse with stress and in the evening. Vomiting does not occur. The neck, back and shoulder muscles in these children are tight and painful. The pain is caused by tight scalp muscles. These tight muscles force the blood out of the scalp. Less blood flow means less oxygen to the tissues and this causes the pain.

Tension headaches often improve with simple pain medications such as Tylenol (acetaminophen), or Advil or Motrin (ibuprofen). Create a calm and pleasant environment. Stressful tasks such as music lessons, sports, and pressure to perform at school may all be causes. Occasionally the child's activity schedule may have to be simplified for a while. Tension headaches may recur and may last, on and off, for years. Tension headaches do not prevent the child from leading a normal life.

Best Advice:

If your child has a headache which persists, check with your doctor.

Hepatitis

Hepatitis is a common viral disease and there are several types.

Hepatitis-A

This is the most common type which children get, often without being very sick. It is spread "stool to mouth." Symptoms are nausea, fatigue, weakness, dark urine, yellow eyeballs and general complaints of not feeling well. After a week or so, the child slowly improves and recovers.

Gamma globulin (a product your doctor has in his or her office) given by injection to others in the household within fourteen days of exposure will prevent infections.

This is also the common form of hepatitis that endangers travelers to foreign, especially Third World, countries. The combination of poor sanitary habits and foods that are not thoroughly cooked makes for a potential risk.

Gamma globulin, injected before travel, will give immunity for three months or more, depending on the dose given. Hepititis-A vacine may also be given.

Hepatitis-B

This is a different virus, spread mainly by blood and body-fluid exchange: sexual contact, intravenous drug use, and blood products. Infected pregnant women may transfer the virus to their babies and infect them. However, 20 to 30 percent of infections have no readily identifiable risk factor, and we do not know how this group becomes infected.

Many people infected with hepatitis-B recover, but a large number become chronic carriers and spread the virus. Eventually chronic hepatitis can cause liver failure. Chronic hepatitis is also the main cause of liver cancer later in life.

Hepatitis-B spreads mainly in the teenage and young adult group. Education against risky behavior such as drug abuse and unprotected sex is important but often has little impact on these activities. An effective and safe vaccine is available and all children (especially teenagers) should get it to protect them against this virulent disease.

Hepatitis-C

This disease is uncommon in children. It probably spreads like hepatitis-B. It is a common cause of chronic liver disease and no vaccine or treatment is available at this time.

Hot weather illnesses/sunburn

The sun is dangerous. Children are more rapidly affected by sun and hot weather because of their small size. Watch your child carefully during the hot summer months.

The sun's ultraviolet rays damage eyes. Sunglasses labeled "UV absorption up to 400 n" or "maximum of 99% UV protection/blockage" or "meets ANSI UV requirements" should be used by one year of age.

Direct and indirect exposure to the sun causes burning of the upper layers of skin or sunburn. The skin becomes red, there is pain, and then blisters form.

Sunburn in childhood has been linked to melanoma, a deadly skin cancer that occurs years later in early to middle adulthood. Other skin cancers that can occur in adults also are due to sun exposure.

Tetracyclines (a type of antibiotic) cause the skin to be more sensitive to sunlight and to burn more rapidly. If your teenager is on one of the tetracyclines for acne, insist that he or she be especially careful.

Preventing sun injury is important: Use a good sunscreen (SPF 15 or more) and cover the child's body with shirts with sleeves, a hat and other protective clothing. Remember to reapply sunscreen after swimming.

For infants use a hypoallergenic sunscreen. Do not apply around the mouth or on the fingers that baby sticks into his or her mouth. Be especially careful to protect your baby from the sun when he or she is in a car seat near a window.

Once skin-burning has occurred, there is little that can be done. Make your child comfortable with cool compresses and Tylenol (acetaminophen).

Heat cramps are pains in the calf or other muscles occurring after strenuous exercise in hot weather. Treat with rest in a cool, shady place and lots of fluids.

More serious are heat exhaustion and heat stroke. To identify and start treatment of either of these conditions you must have a thermometer to measure the child's or teenager's temperature.

Heat exhaustion occurs when the child has sweated out large amounts of fluids and salt and is not drinking enough to replace the fluid. The child is listless, pale or red, may vomit, be dizzy, and pass out. The temperature is elevated, but below 105° F.

Treatment is immediate cooling and lots of fluids. It is important to watch the temperature carefully so that it does not continue to rise. If there is any question, call your doctor. If the temperature comes down, continued intake of fluids and cooling will make the child well.

Heat stroke is an emergency. The temperature is over 105.8° F and rising rapidly. The skin is hot and dry. The child is confused and irritable. Immediate cooling with ice and cold water should be started and fluids given if the child can drink. As soon as possible, transport the child to an emergency room for further treatment.

Permanent brain damage and death may occur if heat stroke is not promptly treated.

Best Advice:

Be respectful of the sun and hot weather. Prevent sunburn to protect your little one from future skin cancer. Give lots of fluids and restrict strenuous activity (especially team sports) in very hot weather. Know where you can easily get hold of a thermometer.

Lyme disease

This is an infectious disease that worries many parents. Lyme disease is caused by a spirochete (borrelia burgdorferi), a germ that when viewed under a microscope shows a corkscrew-like shape. Lyme disease spreads to humans through the bite of a deer tick. These ticks are common on the East Coast but they also live in the woods of the West and Northwest.

Often when a person is infected, a red, circular skin rash forms like a ring around the bite site. This rash grows and may look like a bull's-eye. The rash may last for weeks or months. There are also flu-like symptoms: fever, chills, aching, eye-pain, nausea, vomiting and fatigue. Improvement may be slow. Many infected people develop arthritis, heart problems, or neurologic difficulties. These may occur weeks to months later.

Early diagnosis and treatment with antibiotics shortens the course of the illness, but some late complications may still occur. There is at the moment no good, quick laboratory test for Lyme disease.

Prevention is important: When your children are in the woods or out camping, they should wear long sleeves, long pants, high socks, and use a tick-repellent available at camping, sports and some drugstores.

Ticks are small, and get larger as they fill up with blood. Once attached and sucking blood, an infected tick still takes twenty-four hours or longer to infect your child.

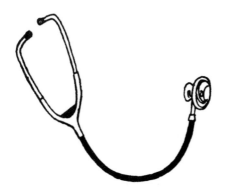

After your family spends time in the woods or camping, inspect your children and yourself for ticks.

There is no surefire way to remove ticks. If a tick is found, carefully pull it out with tweezers and try to get the head out.

Best Advice:

Do not stop camping or other outside activities for fear of Lyme disease; just be careful. Do not panic if you find a tick. Get it out. If worried, check with your doctor.

Nosebleeds

Nosebleeds are common in children. There are many causes for nosebleeds, but the most common is a nasal allergy: The child gets a small area of eczema (dry, crusty irritation) along the middle divider of the nose. The area itches. The child rubs his or her nose, causing the skin to crack, and then bleeding starts.

What *not* to do:

- Do not make the child lie down. That just causes the blood to run down the back of the throat into the stomach.

- Do not apply ice or a cold-water cloth to his or her nose or forehead. That helps very little, if at all.

You can stop almost all nosebleeds by having your child sit up, face forward and nose pointing down. Take a handful of tissues and have your child blow his or her nose. (All the soft clots must be blown out). Then, using your thumb and index finger, pinch your child's nose firmly. Have him or her breathe through the mouth, and do not let go of the child's nose for a minimum of fifteen minutes. This pressure will result in a small, dry, firmly-attached scab, rather than a large, soft clot which will come loose.

To prevent future nosebleeds, put a little Cortaid (.5 percent cortisone) or Cortizone-10 (1 percent cortisone) up each of the child's nostrils. Gently spread it inside the nostrils a few times a day. Do this for a few days, and then you will need to do it only two or three times a week. For the typical allergic nosebleed, this works as well or better than having the nose cauterized.

Pink eye
(conjunctivitis)

Eye infections are common and most children will get them. The cause is either a bacteria or virus. The white of the eye and the inner lids get red and there is drainage of a clear or yellow material. The eye hurts, so the child rubs the face and eye area. This rapidly spreads the infection to the other eye, and to the eyes of brothers, sisters and parents if the hands are not well-washed.

It is usually impossible to distinguish between viral and bacterial pink eye so antibiotic eye-drops are necessary. Pink eye also can be treated with antibiotics taken by mouth.

About 80 percent of infants and toddlers have an ear infection associated with their pink eye. This is why in this age group the child needs to be checked by a doctor. If an ear infection coexists, eye drops alone will not help and antibiotics by mouth are necessary for a cure.

Pneumonia

Viral upper respiratory tract infections (cold and cough) are common in children. Viral infections change the normal state of the lungs and make it easier for bacteria to grow. Viral or bacterial growth spread in the lung itself is called pneumonia.

There are three common types of pneumonia.

Viral pneumonia

Viral infection of the lung frequently causes a pneumonia. There is a cold and cough for several days and then the pneumonia starts. The peak years for viral pneumonia are two to three years of age. Most viral pneumonias are caused by RSV, parainfluenza viruses, adenoviruses or enteroviruses.

There is often a cough and there may be some rapid or difficult breathing. The child's temperature may vary and he or she may not appear very ill. Viral pneumonia may be difficult to differentiate from bacterial or mycoplasma pneumonia. Antibiotics do not help. Treatment consists of fever control, the humidifier, an expectorant cough medicine and waiting it out.

Bacterial pneumonia

This commonly follows viral infections of the lung. The most common bacterial cause for pneumonia is the pneumococcus. Sudden fever, chills and a cough, which are common in older children, may be absent in infants and toddlers.

Usually there is a cough and low grade fever which then suddenly goes up to 103° F or more. The child may appear quite ill (see How to Tell if Your Child is Really Ill, page 21). The white blood count is elevated and there will be changes on the chest X-ray. Treatment consists of antibiotics. If the child is older and not too sick, treatment at home, rather than at a hospital, is certainly possible.

Mycoplasma pneumonia

Mycoplasma is an organism which is not a virus but also is not a true bacterium (it is somewhere in between). Mycoplasma is a frequent cause of bronchitis and pneumonia in children, and especially teenagers. This is what used to be called walking pneumonia. The child or teenager may not be very ill and often continues with normal activity, though he or she is tired and coughing. This infection can last for several weeks before it becomes better on its own. Treatment with erythromycin, an antibiotic, usually rapidly makes mycoplasma pneumonia better.

Best Advice:

Pneumonias are fairly common in children. They are usually caused by virus infections and usually are not too serious. Any child who looks ill, with a cough and high fever, should be seen by the doctor.

Poison oak, ivy and sumac

This nasty rash is spread by direct contact with the plant, and in susceptible children can be a real nuisance.

Prevention is important. Put long-sleeved shirts and long pants on your child when he or she is going through or playing in thick vegetation.

Once the child's skin has the red spots and blisters, it is important to wash the child and all of his or her clothes, so that there is no further spreading of the rash.

A mild cortisone cream (Cortaid) helps to control the itching, as does Benadryl (diphenhydramine hydrochloride), an antihistamine taken by mouth. Both can be purchased over-the-counter at your drugstore. Once the rash and itch start, the process continues for two to five days or so, even with treatment. In severe cases, oral steroid medications prescribed by your doctor may be necessary.

Splinters

Children often get splinters under their skin, especially in the summer when they are playing outdoors. Most splinter wounds are superficial with the splinter lodged in the upper outer layer of skin of the hands or feet.

If part of the splinter sticks out, it is easily removed. If it is visible under the skin and bothersome for the child, a sterile needle or safety-pin (heat the tip in a flame until it is red hot to kill all the bacteria) will help you tease most splinters out.

Deep splinters do occur. They are painful and the child will let you know that something is wrong. If the deep splinter has a part that sticks out, very carefully try to pull it out, in the direction that the splinter entered. You don't want to break it and leave the tip behind.

If it comes out and seems to be in one piece, soak the area in hot soapy water for some time and apply an antibiotic ointment (Neosporin or Polysporin). Soak several times a day for a few days and watch for infection. Make sure your child's tetanus shots are up to date (see also Immunizations, page 15). If the area becomes red and swollen, probably part of the splinter was left behind and a visit to the doctor is necessary. Occasionally the splinter is so deep that it is impossible to get it all out. Soaking the area in hot soapy water several times a day is the treatment of choice. Most of the time the broken-off part migrates to the surface and comes out on its own after some days or weeks.

Best Advice:

Splinters are common and most of the time not a problem. If a piece of the splinter breaks off in the child, soaking often helps. Occasionally the doctor does have to find and pull out the broken-off piece, or start the child on antibiotics for infection.

Teeth, injuries to

Teeth often get injured during the growing years. The child falls and hits an object or has something hard in the mouth when the injury occurs. This can loosen teeth, push them into the gums or knock them out.

Most injured, loose baby teeth reattach themselves and end up fine.

Many injured teeth look normal at first but later turn a dark color. This means that the tooth has died. Dead baby teeth remain in place most of the time and are perfectly functional. They act as spacers for the teeth that will follow and should be left alone. Occasionally the tooth will become infected. A "gum boil," a small, painless red bump, draining pus, will appear on the gum above the tooth. If that happens your dentist will prescribe an antibiotic and recommend that the tooth be pulled.

If the injury is enough to completely knock out the tooth, especially if it is a permanent tooth, find the tooth and immediately call your dentist. In the meantime, the ideal place to keep the tooth is in saliva (spit), in your mouth if the child is small or in the child's mouth if he or she is old enough not to swallow the tooth. Most dentists know how to reimplant the tooth into the gum. This should save the tooth.

Best Advice:

Tooth injuries are common and usually turn out all right. It is best to check with your dentist if the teeth do not look the way they should, if loose, or if the tooth is out and you have it.

Tuberculosis

Tuberculosis is a bacterial infection that had been almost wiped out in the United States until recent years. Currently it is on the rise.

Tuberculosis is a potentially serious infection which spreads from one person to another
through coughing. The person spreading the
disease must have an open lesion (cavity) in his
lung to spread the TB germs. Once the TB bacteria enter the child's lung the bacteria settle in
and are contained by the child's immune system. A wall of fibrous material forms around the
bacteria. This prevents the bacteria from
spreading through the body. The bacteria remain dormant, but alive, indefinitely.

Any time that there are live TB bacteria in
the body, the TB skin test (PPD) turns positive
after about six weeks and remains positive. It is
an excellent screening test to see who has been
infected.

Clinically the child feels fine, is not contagious, and there are no symptoms. This is called
primary tuberculosis. The chest X-ray will be
normal and the diagnosis is made with the TB
skin test (see PPD, page 19). To ensure that these
TB bacteria remain contained, your doctor will
treat your child with anti-TB medication (by
mouth) for six to nine months. Your child is not
contagious during this time and should continue
to lead a normal life.

The source of the infection is frequently a
family member with a chronic cough who is in
close contact with the child. If your child has
primary TB, the entire family should be screened
with a TB test or chest X-rays. Often the infected

person cannot be found. Then it has to be assumed that the child was exposed away from the home.

Rarely, if there are many bacteria inhaled and the resistance of the child is low, an active, spreading infection starts. A pneumonia forms (changes are seen on the chest X-ray) and the child will be clinically ill with fever, weight loss and listlessness. This is called active tuberculosis. In children under 13, lung cavities occur infrequently and most, even with active disease, are not contagious. From the lung, the TB germ can spread to the bones, brain or anywhere in the body. Rest and treatment for many months with antibiotics works well to cure this disease.

Best Advice:

If your child has a positive skin test for TB, it is not the end of the world. Probably your child will have primary TB, will take medication by mouth and will continue to lead a normal life.

Sprains and strains

Joint and bone injuries are common in children. Remember: "RICE" (Rest, Ice, Compression, Elevation). Apply ice and compress by wrapping with an Ace bandage. Alternate between icing and compression every thirty minutes. This helps for the first forty-eight hours. After that, heat helps. If pain persists, if there is severe swelling, or if it just looks wrong, there may be a broken bone. Call your doctor.

Swimmer's ear
(external otitis)

Swimmer's ear is an infection of the ear canal. It is caused by water left in the ear after swimming and is common in the summer months. Try to prevent the infection by rinsing the child's ears out with a mixture of rubbing alcohol and white vinegar:

To one pint bottle of rubbing alcohol add two to three tablespoons of white vinegar. When your child comes out of the water, rinse both ears out with this mixture. Fill the ear to the brim, then let the mixture run back out. The alcohol/white vinegar mixture picks up the water and, as it evaporates, leaves the ear canal dry.

If your child has an earache, especially one that gets worse as you pull on the outer ear, all swimming must stop. Rinse the ears out three or four times a day with white vinegar. If this does not help after a few days, see your doctor.

Testicular pain

Testicular pain in boys is common after injuries. There may be some swelling and redness. Rest, ice and a good support are usually all that is necessary. Preteens and teenagers also can get pain in their testes from infections. There is slowly progressive swelling, moderate tenderness and redness of the sack. Often antibiotics are needed and a visit to your doctor is necessary.

This age group also may get something called testicular torsion. The testicle hangs on a cord, and if it is not attached solidly in the scrotum (sack) it will twist on itself on the cord. This cuts off the blood supply to the testicle. Typically the boy complains of sudden, sharp, unrelenting pain in the testicle. The involved side of the sack rapidly becomes swollen, red and hard. It may occur during or after exercise, during sleep, or at any time. If the testicle is not untwisted to allow blood to flow back into it, the testicle dies. This can happen within a few hours after the pain starts.

If your boy complains of sudden, severe testicular pain it is a true emergency. Call your doctor to have the boy seen immediately, or go to an emergency room. The testicle must be surgically untwisted to save it.

Testicular tumors

Tumors of the testicle are painless lumps which grow slowly. Testicular tumors are often malignant, but are easily felt because of their location, and the cure rate is excellent if found early. They are most common in the teen years and early twenties. Any testicular lump must be immediately checked by your doctor. When your boy enters puberty ask your doctor to show him how to examine his testicles monthly. This is good preventive medicine.

Vomiting and diarrhea (Gastroenteritis)

Gastroenteritis, an inflammation of the lining of the stomach and intestine, usually starts with a bellyache, vomiting and/or diarrhea. There may be a little fever and other flu-like symptoms.

If your child is not vomiting and has only loose bowel movements, continue feeding him or her a bland diet and encourage him or her to drink lots of fluids. The symptoms often stop after several days and the child will feel well again.

If vomiting starts, stop everything and give very small quantities (one to two teaspoons) of clear fluids every fifteen minutes. You can use de-fizzed soda, Gatorade, apple juice, Popsicles or buy Pedialyte or Ricelyte at the drugstore. Classic Coca Cola with the fizz taken out often stops vomiting when nothing else will. As soon as the vomiting stops, start small quantities of bland foods—very small amounts—at frequent intervals.

Best Advice:

Most gastroenteritis can be safely handled at home. It is better to give a teaspoon of fluid to a vomiting child and have it stay down, than to give an ounce and have it come back up.

If the vomiting continues, or if your child looks ill, then it is time to call your doctor.

Warts

Warts, which are caused by viruses, are common. Almost every child will have a few warts at some time or another. Warts may be unsightly and embarrass the child.

- Warts spread through contact, and increase in number if irritated.

- Plain warts are usually on the fingers, hands, elbows and knees.

- Flat warts occur on the face and neck.

- Plantar warts are on the soles of the feet.

All warts are self-limiting: They always go away by themselves, but it may take several years.

Warts are harmless. They never cause cancer or other serious problems. However, plantar warts may be painful as they are hard and walking on one is like walking on any hard object.

A dermatologist can remove warts with liquid nitrogen, which freezes them. This is quite effective, but expensive.

Any of a multitude of wart medicines available over-the-counter at the drugstore will cause a wart to disappear.

(See also Wart medications, page 180)

Best Advice:

Warts are harmless. If you do nothing, they always eventually go away.

Eighteen

Your Child and Medicines

There will be times when you will have medications for your child, either prescribed by your doctor or bought at the drugstore without a prescription. Here are some important facts you should know:

Antibiotics

These medications are used when your child has a bacterial infection. Antibiotics are substances that mimic natural nutrients that bacteria use. The antibiotic enters the blood stream, the bacteria think it is food, and try to use it to grow and multiply. Once inside the bacteria, some antibiotics actually destroy them. These antibiotics are fast-acting and very efficient. Other antibiotics do not kill the bacteria but prevent them from multiplying. This then allows the body's natural defenses to mobilize and kill the bacteria. These antibiotics are not quite as efficient, but for practical purposes work almost as well.

If your child is sick with a bacterial infection, but the bacteria do not use the nutrient that the prescribed antibiotic mimics, the antibiotic will not work. A different one is needed. This does not mean that the first antibiotic does not work in your child, only that the bacteria causing this infection were not sensitive to it. The same antibiotic may work well with the next illness, when other bacteria are the cause.

Antibiotics do not kill viruses and should not be used for viral infections.

Every time an antibiotic is used, it kills the weaker bacteria first. The hardier ones take longer to die. If the antibiotic is stopped too soon, these hardier bacteria, having survived, may become used to this particular antibiotic. The next time the antibiotic is used, it may not work. It is therefore important that your child takes all of the prescribed antibiotic. That will prevent the hardier bacteria from surviving and causing future resistant infections.

As different infections need different antibiotics, your doctor can not really prescribe one without seeing the child. It is NOT good medicine to get antibiotic prescriptions over the telephone.

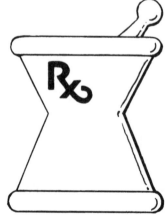

Best Advice:

Do not ask your doctor to prescribe anti-biotics without seeing your child.

Always be certain your child finishes ALL the antibiotic prescribed, even if he or she is well before the prescription is completely used.

Generic drugs

Generic drugs are "copies" of brand-name drugs produced and tested by drug companies and approved for use by the responsible government agencies. As generics do not need new research or testing, they are usually cheaper than the "original." The only requirement is that they are chemically the same. They may not look like the "real thing" and may not taste as good. Most generics, including antibiotics, work about as well as the researched and tested drug. We do know that some heart and epilepsy generics, though chemically the same as the original, do not work as well in the body.

If your insurance company mandates generics, ask your doctor to make sure that the substituted drug works adequately.

Best Advice:

If your pharmacist gives you a generic medication, make sure a generic is what your doctor ordered.

Medication expiration dates

All medications, by law, must have an expiration date. It implies that the medication is no longer good after that date. This is true for liquid antibiotics mixed by your pharmacist. It is also true for tetracycline antibiotics in capsule or pill form. Almost everything else—cough medications, antihistamines, asthma medications and ointments—though they may lose a little of their potency, for practical purposes remain good for a long time after the listed date.

With the high cost of medications, do not throw recently outdated drugs away. If your doctor changes medication, keep the leftover pills or capsules (except tetracyclines) in the refrigerator in child-proof containers. Check with your doctor to see if you can use the same medication later on if needed.

Nineteen

Common Medications

Here are some of the common medications you may need. You can buy most of them at the drugstore without a prescription.

Fever and/or pain medications

Analgesics and antipyretics are medications used to treat pain and to lower the temperature if there is a fever.

In years past, aspirin would have been recommended for children to relieve fever or pain, but it is now associated with Reyes syndrome, a rare but deadly disease of the liver and brain and should not be given to children.

Acetaminophen is a common analgesic/antipyretic. Common brand names are Tylenol, Tempra, and Liquiprin. These all come in infant drops, teaspoon and chewable form. They are all interchangeable. Adult tablets are available. Generic brands are available.

Another common analgesic/antipyretic is ibuprofen. Children's Advil, liquid, and children's Motrin, liquid and chewable, are brands of ibuprofen.

Children's Advil is available by prescription only at this time. Tablets for older children and teenagers are available without a prescription. Generic brands are available in tablets.

For teenagers naproxen sodium is available as Aleve brand tablets without a prescription.

Cold medications

These are usually antihistamines, decongestants or a combination of both. These products dry up the nose and help control sneezing.

Chlor-Trimeton (chlorpheniramine maleate), and diphenhydramine hydrochloride are antihistamines. They dry up noses and help control itching. Benadryl is a commonly available brand of diphenhydramine hydrochloride.

Pseudoephedrine is a decongestant. It will dry up the nose and not make the child drowsy (good if the child has to go to school). Sudafed is a common brand name of pseudoephedrine.

Triaminic (all colors), Pedia Care, Rondec, Dimetapp, Naldecon are brand name decongestant and antihistamine combinations, are interchangeable and work fairly well.

Many of the cold medications also come with the analgesic/antipyretic acetaminophen already added. It is not a good idea to use these combinations. If your child has pain or a fever along with the cold, use your cold medication and give acetaminophen (Tylenol) separately. This way you can better control the dose that you need to use for each drug.

Cough medications

Doctors usually recommend expectorants.

These loosen mucus and help the child to cough it up, rather than stopping the cough.

Robitussin (all) and Tussi-Organidin are brand name expectorants that work very well.

If you need a nighttime medication to suppress the cough, you can use Delsym.

Phenergan expectorant with codeine is very good, but you will need a prescription.

Degasser and antacid medications

These medications decrease gas and may make bellyaches feel better.

Simethicone is recommended for colic. Phazyme or Mylicon drops are two brands of simethicone and are interchangeable.

Name brands Maalox Plus and Mylanta contain an antacid along with simethicone. Both come as tablets and liquid and often help reduce abdominal pain and/or gas in older children.

Cuts and abrasion medications

Neosporin and Polysporin are brand name antibiotic ointments (a combination of polymyxin B sulfate, bacitracin zinc, and neomycin) which work well for skin infections resulting from cuts and abrasions.

Fungus medications

Clotrimazole and miconazole ointments

work well for yeast and other fungal infections. Lotrimin is a brand name for clotrimazole and Micatin is a brand of miconazole.

Allergy medications

Anti-inflammatory medications Cortaid (.5 percent cortisone) and Cortizone 10 (1 percent cortisone) work well for eczema, dry skin, and other allergic rashes.

Diphenhydramine hydrochloride, an anti-histamine available under the brand name Benadryl, works very well for itching and also makes the child sleepy. This is a good medicine to use when your child itches and is miserable with ailments such as chicken pox, insect stings, and poison ivy.

Acne medications

Benzoyl peroxide, available in ointment form as Oxy-5, Oxy-10, Clearasil and other brand names, works fairly well as do the same brands' antibiotic (triclosan) soaps. Both the ointment and soap (use both) are worth a trial before you spend more on prescription medications.

Wart medications

Compound-W and DuoFilm are two brands of medication that work as well as anything to get rid of warts, except actual removal of the wart by a doctor.

What to Include in a Household First-Aid Kit

Every home should have a box or shelf (preferably with a child-proof door) to keep some basic medications. Include the following:

- A list of emergency information (see page 184)

- Adhesive strip bandages (Band-Aids)

- Cotton balls

- Cotton swabs

- Safety pins

- Thermometer (glass-mercury or electronic for oral or rectal use)

- Antibiotic ointment: Neosporin or Polysporin for open scrapes, small cuts or small burns

- An antifungal ointment: Micatin for diaper rash, athlete's foot or jock-strap itch

- An expectorant cough medicine: Robitussin-DM for when your child has a cough

- A nasal decongestant (Triaminic, Dimetapp or Sudafed): to use for colds and allergies

- An antihistamine (Benadryl, liquid and capsules): for hives, allergies and insect bites

- An antacid/degasser (Maalox Plus): for mild stomachaches

- Liquid analgesic/antipyretic (Tylenol liquid): for pain and/or fever with smaller children

- Analgesic/antipyretic tablets (Tylenol): for pain and/or fever with older children and adults

- Syrup of ipecac, 1 ounce size: causes vomiting in case of poisoning. Do NOT use without checking with your doctor or the Poison Control Center.

- One 2-inch wide and one 4-inch wide Ace bandage (elastic bandage) for sprained ankles.

Recommended Hours of Sleep— Infants, Children, Teenagers

Age	Night Hours	Nap Hours	Total Hours
1 wk-1 mo	8-9	8	16-17
6 mo	10	4	14
9 mo-2 yr	11-12	2-3	13-15
3 yr	10	2	12
5 yr	11	0	11
9 yr	10	0	10
14 yr	9	0	9
16 yr	7-9	0	7-9
18 yr	7-8	0	7-8

Sleep time varies. Some children need more sleep than others. If you worry about the amount of time your child sleeps, call your doctor.

Emergency Information

Emergency Phone Numbers

Fire: _____

Police: _____

Ambulance: _____

Poison Control Center: _____

Animal Control: _____

Doctor

Name: _____

Address: _____

Phone: _____

Hospital

Name: _____

Address: _____

Phone: _____

Mom's work phone: _____

Dad's work phone: _____

Neighbors, Friends and Relatives

Name: _____

Phone: _____

Name: _____

Phone: _____

Instructions: *Photocopy this page twice, fill out both copies, and post one on the side of the refrigerator or other easy-to-find spot—be sure to point it out to your baby-sitters—and place the other copy with your first-aid supplies.*

**The Pediatrician's
New Baby Owner's Manual**

Family Health History

Genetics play a significant part in our overall health. Record here any major health problems, such as diabetes, heart disease or cancer, experienced by family members and share this information with your doctor. Be sure to update this information from time to time.

_____

Paternal Grandfather

Name: _____

Paternal Grandmother

Name: _____

Family Health History

Maternal Grandfather

Name: _____

Maternal Grandmother

Name: _____

Family Health History

Dad

Name: _____

Mom

Name: _____

Family Health History

Child

Name: _____

Child

Name: _____

Family Health History

Child

Name: _____

Child

Name: _____

Family Health History

Child

Name: _____

Child

Name: _____

Index

Index

Index

Index

Trademark Information

About the Author

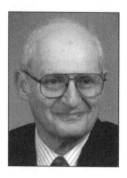

Horst D. Weinberg, M.D., received his M.D. degree from the University of Chicago School of Medicine. He is the host of Central California's popular weekly call-in TV program "The Doctor is In."

He has been a frequent contributor to such journals as *The American Journal of Diseases of Children*, *Contemporary Pediatrics* and the *Western Journal of Medicine*.

Dr. Weinberg's awards include the Distinguished Achievement Award from the American Heart Association and the Special Resident Teaching Award from Central California's Valley Children's Hospital.

Dr. Weinberg has been a pediatrician for over forty years. He lives with his wife Carol in Fresno, California. They have three grown children.

**To order additional copies
of this book, please call
1-800-497-4909
or write to
Quill Driver Books
8386 N. Madsen
Clovis, CA 93611.
Credit cards accepted.**